D0829627

Prostate Cancer Survivors Speak Their Minds

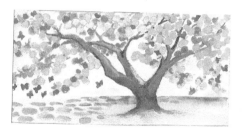

In Search of a Cure

Donated by

Anne M. & Joel L. Pearl

Prostate Cancer Survivors Speak Their Minds

Advice on Options, Treatments, and Aftereffects

Arthur L. Burnett II, M.D.,
and Norman S. Morris

WILEY

John Wiley & Sons, Inc.

Copyright © 2010 by Arthur L. Burnett II, and Norman S. Morris. All rights reserved

Published by John Wiley & Sons, Inc., Hoboken, New Jersey
Published simultaneously in Canada

No part of this publication may be reproduced, stored in a retrieval system, or transmitted in any form or by any means, electronic, mechanical, photocopying, recording, scanning, or otherwise, except as permitted under Section 107 or 108 of the 1976 United States Copyright Act, without either the prior written permission of the Publisher, or authorization through payment of the appropriate per-copy fee to the Copyright Clearance Center, 222 Rosewood Drive, Danvers, MA 01923, (978) 750-8400, fax (978) 646-8600, or on the web at www.copyright.com. Requests to the Publisher for permission should be addressed to the Permissions Department, John Wiley & Sons, Inc., 111 River Street, Hoboken, NJ 07030, (201) 748-6011, fax (201) 748-6008, or online at http://www.wiley.com/go/permissions.

The information contained in this book is not intended to serve as a replacement for professional medical advice. Any use of the information in this book is at the reader's discretion. The author and the publisher specifically disclaim any and all liability arising directly or indirectly from the use or application of any information contained in this book. A health care professional should be consulted regarding your specific situation.

For general information about our other products and services, please contact our Customer Care Department within the United States at (800) 762-2974, outside the United States at (317) 572-3993 or fax (317) 572-4002.

Wiley also publishes its books in a variety of electronic formats. Some content that appears in print may not be available in electronic books. For more information about Wiley products, visit our web site at www.wiley.com.

Library of Congress Cataloging-in-Publication Data:
Burnett, Arthur.
  Prostate cancer survivors speak their minds: advice on options, treatments, and aftereffects/Arthur L. Burnett II and Norman S. Morris.
       p. cm.
  Includes bibliographical references and index.
  ISBN 978-0470-57881-0 (pbk)
  ISBN 978-0470-64211-5 (special edition)
  ISBN 978-0470-62091-5 (ebk)
  ISBN 978-0470-62101-1 (ebk)
  ISBN 978-0470-62102-8 (ebk)
  1. Prostate–Cancer. 2. Prostate–Cancer–Patients. I. Morris, Norman S. II. Title.
  RC280.P7B874 2010
  616.99'463—dc22

                                                                    2009051015

Printed in the United States of America

10 9 8 7 6 5 4 3 2 1

For Sandy and Rhonice. They have graced our lives with love, encouragement, and devotion.

—Norman and Bud

For my late brother, Myron, physician, humanist, philanthropist, and advocate for the needy and infirm.

—Norman

Contents

Prescriptive Information

For your quick reference, below are informational sections you can go to immediately.

Foreword

By Senator John Kerry

If you're opening this book, you or a loved one are probably among the millions of us who got a diagnosis you probably never expected: prostate cancer.

It's jarring. And it's scary.

I guess I always told myself I was pretty indestructible. I'd been in combat as a young man. I'd been face-to-face with some hardened criminals as a prosecutor in Massachusetts. But in 2002, just as I was beginning my campaign to be president of the United States, I faced a very different kind of challenge—I was diagnosed with prostate cancer. The words hit like a swift kick to the midsection. I was no stranger to cancer, but like anyone else, hearing the word in the same breath as my own name was something I'd never anticipated. Years ago my grandfather died of colon cancer, and in the year 2000 I watched my father, in his eighties, struggle with prostate cancer. This was a battle he too would lose.

My family members' cancers were caught too late, and from these experiences I learned the importance of early testing. In addition, I was lucky to be married to the daughter of a doctor and to have a daughter in medical school. They both consistently reminded me to get tested.

But nothing fully prepares you for that diagnosis.

With the help of my family, friends, and doctors—and the best health care on earth—I beat prostate cancer. I picked myself up and went on. I was lucky.

I learned a lot from my bout with cancer. I learned a little more humility. I learned how many people would get the same diagnosis and wouldn't end up healthy like me because they didn't have good health insurance.

I also learned that when you get that diagnosis you instantly join a fraternity of people you never before realized you were linked to. Bob Dole called me in the hospital. Hamilton Jordan called me. And so did Lance Armstrong. No politics, just people who wanted to help—and to share their wisdom and their example.

That's partly what makes this book special: simply by having battled and survived cancer we are now part of a second "Band of Brothers," and together we'd like to do what we can to help others going through the same scare.

So, given a choice between being scared of cancer and being philosophical about it, I'd rather just be pissed off at cancer and use my anger to do what I like to do—be an advocate and help those who are going through the same thing. What cancer did was open my eyes even more to what was going on around me, and make me that much more determined to help others who aren't as lucky as I was. Survivorship isn't just grace or relief. It comes with responsibility to help others.

And there's a hell of a lot of work to do. According to the American Cancer Society (ACS), in 2008, there were 186,320 new cases of prostate cancer and 28,660 deaths as a result. Prostate cancer is also the most frequently diagnosed cancer and the leading cause of cancer death in men. On a more positive note, more than 90 percent of prostate cancer is diagnosed in what is known as the "local and regional stages" and correlates to an almost 100 percent survival rate in the first five years.

Unfortunately, these gains haven't been shared by all Americans. Significant disparities remain. Mortality rates are more than twice as high among African American men. The closer you look, the more disconcerting the facts become. According to the American Cancer Society's report for African Americans for

2007–2008, black men have a 60 percent higher average annual rate of prostate cancer than white men do. Fewer black men diagnose their cancer early, despite the fact that the ACS recommends that African American men begin annual prostate cancer screening starting between the ages of forty and forty-five.

We need to raise awareness. That—again—is why books like *Prostate Cancer Survivors Speak Their Minds* are so important. A long, long time ago I adopted a personal philosophy after a different kind of struggle: "Every day is extra." My brush with cancer left me feeling that the best way to truly beat cancer is to make the most of those "extra days"—to live as fully and as fearlessly as I possibly can. Not just to live as if I'd never had the cancer, but to live with the wisdom and resolve I gained from beating it.

Dr. Arthur L. Burnett II, director of Johns Hopkins's Male Consultation Clinic and one of the leading authorities on prostate cancer, along with Norman Morris, Emmy Award–winning journalist and producer with CBS News and prostate cancer survivor, have written a terrific, thoughtful, and eye-opening book. Before they were coauthors, Burnett and Morris teamed up on another endeavor: curing Norman Morris's prostate cancer.

Their work will help to bridge the gap between doctor and patient, between science and emotion, and between surviving and living. Let's hope that the personal stories detailed throughout this book will help to save the lives of those diagnosed—and those not yet diagnosed—with prostate cancer.

I hope that this book, and maybe even the little I have shared about my own experience, will help you or a loved one in your own fight—along with terrific doctors, some prayer, a tremendous amount of support from family and friends, and a little luck.

Prostate Cancer Survivors Speak Their Minds is not just an argument for beating cancer by living life fully—it's also a testament to one man's triumph and the brilliant doctor who made it possible.

John Kerry is the chairman of the Senate Foreign Relations Committee and was the 2004 Democratic candidate for president of the United States.

Acknowledgments

Bill Moyers once told me that if you get in a car and drive across America you will have a book. My late and good friend Studs Terkel, one of the country's great oral historians, told me the same thing. And when Studs found out I was a prostate cancer survivor, he urged me to go across America and write a book that could help patients better understand the complex disease they were dealing with and so enable them to decide a course of action that would save their lives. The idea excited me. To help just one man make the most important decision in his life was enough to motivate me, but to reach out and help thousands who are diagnosed with prostate cancer represented a challenge I was certainly up for. When I mentioned the project to my surgeon, Dr. Arthur Burnett, he told me not to proceed without him. And so our partnership came to pass.

Trusted friends rallied around. Van Gordon Sauter, former president of CBS News, and Jim Houtrides, a former CBS News senior producer, and his wife, Maureen, were quick to offer encouragement. Bruce Lee, former senior editor of Morrow Books, believed in our mission and showed us the way. Then there were the earthmovers: my wife, Sandy, the sunshine of my life and a wielder of a nasty editing pen; Whitney Erickson, a vice president of American Medical Systems, whose incredible support and backing made our work possible; and Evalyn Lee Bacon, a protégé at CBS News and now a trusted friend, who helped keep me focused at difficult moments.

Thanks and appreciation go to many others, principally to Dr. Arnon Krongrad of the Krongrad Institute in Aventura, Florida, and Dr. Neil Sherman of the UMDNJ Urology Department in Newark, New Jersey, for offering the names of patients in this book with important stories to tell, and to Dr. Burnett's tireless assistant, Debbie Lassen, for her contributions.

We, of course, reserve our heartfelt thanks to all the patients whose voices are heard in this book, who along with their wives and partners took the time and effort to share the most intimate details of their lives so that others can benefit.

Finally, we applaud all those fine folks behind the scene who make a book like this a reality. A curtain call please for our agent, Faith Hamlin, for her extraordinary work and patience with the authors; for the Wiley editorial team, led by Tom Miller and his right hand, Christel Winkler; and for the marketing, promotion, and sales workaholics whom few of us ever see. Thank you.

Introduction

If you are a person of a certain age, you may remember some secret words that adults didn't want you to know. One I recall was the C word. In whispers, my mother would tell a friend or relative that Uncle Harry died of "C." When I was growing up you couldn't pry that mystery out of any member of the family. Even the letter "C" conjured up some sort of chamber of horrors. Finally, somebody uttered the word aloud and the genie was out of the bottle.

Today, we throw that C word around without the trepidation of our parents. Cancer is still an ugly word, but here is the good news. More and more, many cancers *can* be cured or controlled. One in particular, prostate cancer, is the focus of this book. Now, caught early enough, the chance that prostate cancer can be "cured" is high. There are caveats, of course, since we are not dealing with an uncomplicated disease, and outcomes from different treatments can vary widely. But the indisputable fact is that over the past several years, though the reported annual incidence of prostate cancer has been rising in the United States, the death rate among prostate cancer patients has been declining due to early diagnosis, constantly improved treatments, and new research.

The aim of this book is not to serve as a medical text, although the reader may want to know some basic facts about prostate cancer treatments. I hope the explanations offered will give meaning and context to the tales prostate patients tell. These are personal and intimate stories told by courageous men. In one way or another, the individual accounts are as unique as the men who relate them. But there is a common theme. As varied as the men may be, they all speak as one in revealing an optimistic view of life despite what they have gone through or continue to experience. They offer inspiration and hope to the many thousands of men who are now dealing with or will later be compelled to face the dreaded enemy called prostate cancer.

Until about a dozen years ago, "prostate" was not a word in my vocabulary. I was running around covering the news for CBS, and I simply had no time to deal with things like personal health issues. When I was not working, I was at home, helping my wife raise three young boys. There was little time left over to concern myself with much else.

My brush with prostate cancer came surreptitiously, a deadly insurgent, waiting silently for the appropriate moment to attack. It would not be an easy fight, but one I was determined to wage. That is true of the men in this book, and it linked all of us as comrades in a battle against a common enemy. Moreover, it made possible the sharing of stories and otherwise private experiences that we hope will give comfort and encouragement to the many who are facing prostate cancer today. The battles go on. The prospects for survival and good outcomes are excellent and are getting better every day!

The coauthor of this book, Dr. Arthur L. Burnett II, is the Patrick C. Walsh Professor of Urology, Cellular and Molecular Medicine at the Brady Urological Institute at the Johns Hopkins Medical Institutions in Baltimore. Dr. Burnett, one of the world's distinguished authorities on prostate cancer, is also director of the Male Consultation Clinic at Hopkins; director of the Hopkins Basic Science Laboratory; director of Neuro-Urology Research; professor of urology and surgery at the Hopkins Medical School; and visiting professor and lecturer on prostate cancer worldwide. He is also renowned for his studies in nitric oxide that led to the discovery of Viagra.

In his role as professor and surgeon at Johns Hopkins, Dr. Burnett exemplifies the highest surgical prostate and urological skills and training in the world. He is the man charged with overseeing this book and forestalling any medical misstatements it might otherwise contain. Dr. Burnett is an exacting taskmaster. He provides his own perspective on each patient's case, helping to frame the story with an objective and accurate medical appraisal of the interviewee's comments.

What You Should Know about Prostate Cancer

Generally, prostate cancer in men under forty-five is rare but can occur, and the risk goes up as a man grows older. On average it attacks men fifty-five or over. But among African American men, the incidence of prostate cancer is 1.5 times higher than in the white male population, and the mortality rate is double. Their incidence is 2.7 times higher than among Asian Americans, who the National Cancer Institute reports have the lowest incidence of prostate cancer in the country, along with Native Americans.

Precise causes for the disparity between black and white men are not known, but the suspected causes are lack of knowledge about the disease, less access to the health-care system, and financial deprivation. Some have pointed out that black men in Africa don't appear to have the disproportionate incidence of prostate cancer that African American men do. But there are major problems in attempting to draw such statistical conclusions. Epidemiological studies in Africa may be flawed. In addition to poor longitudinal studies, there is simply poor accuracy in African cancer statistics. Because of the high prevalence of AIDS, many men don't survive long enough to acquire the diagnosis.

The latest comprehensive report released by the U.S. Department of Health and Human Services shows that, aside from skin cancers, prostate cancer is the leading cancer affecting men of all races in the United States. Progress has been made in treating prostate cancer. About one man in six will be diagnosed with prostate cancer during his lifetime, but only one man in thirty-five will die of it! Today, more than two million men in the United States who were treated at some point are still alive. That represents significant progress.

In the late 1990s, there was a surge of newly diagnosed cases of prostate cancer due principally to the introduction and widespread use of a new detection tool called the prostate-specific antigen (PSA) test. The PSA is a blood test that can detect the possible presence of prostate cancer. Over the last decade, advances in detection and treatment (including radical prostatectomies, radiation interventions, and hormone suppression) have done much to reduce mortality rates. Given all the strides in dealing with prostate cancer cases, the number of annual cases and the instances of death from prostate cancer appear, at present, to have reached a plateau. But the aging baby boomer generation is certain to raise both annual incidence levels and mortality rates. Early detection and intervention offer the promise of survival, but truthfully, there will be instances in this aging population where the discovery of prostate cancer will be at a late stage. So it is expected that incidence and mortality levels will one day plateau again, but at higher levels. A dramatic reduction in mortality rates from prostate cancer awaits the arrival of stunning new research and modes of discovery and intervention that we hope will one day appear.

On the following pages you will find stories from men who have encountered the enemy, and some who are still in the line of fire. You will find heterosexuals and gays, married men and bachelors, working men and retired, celebrities and ordinary people, and finally their wives, lovers, and partners. There is much to learn from their revelations. Some readers may come to identify with accounts or incidents that to a degree mirror their own issues or experiences, perhaps assisting them in the difficult process of making critical decisions.

Treatments and Decisions

It can't be said often enough: *When it comes to selecting treatment, one size does not fit all*, whether the treatment be surgery, external beam therapy (radiation), seed implants, cryotherapy, expectant management, pharmacology, or herbal remedy. From a medical standpoint, the decision should properly be made on the patient's physical condition and psychological preference. Still, the final choice is the patient's, and for whatever reason, the patient may elect to accept or reject a physician's recommendations.

Today, radical prostatectomy is referred to as the "gold standard" for the treatment of early-stage prostate cancer. That certainly wasn't always true. A mere twenty years ago, surgery carried high risks of postoperative complications, including decreased physical capacity, long-term incontinence, and permanent erectile dysfunction. Clinical surveys have shown that postoperative erectile function is of profound importance to patients.

It took landmark research, beginning in the 1980s, and the subsequent development of new surgical techniques by Johns Hopkins's past chief urology surgeon, Dr. Patrick Walsh, and his associates to completely change the landscape of erectile dysfunction. Their work led to the discovery of the basis for preserving erectile function following radical prostatectomy. The technique involves the preservation of the cavernous nerves and is now known simply as "nerve sparing."

Nerve sparing is now practiced at major academic centers and is performed by highly trained and experienced surgeons. Satisfactory recovery for sexual function following surgery at these centers ranges between 60 and 85 percent. Results are acknowledged to vary at different institutions. Ninety-five percent of men who have undergone nerve-sparing prostatectomies at Johns Hopkins have achieved full urinary continence—meaning no pads—in two to six months after surgery.

Does the fact that radical prostatectomy is the gold standard for curing prostate cancer mean that surgery is best for every patient? Dr. Burnett's response is a resounding no! Age, physical condition, and other preexisting risk factors enter into the equation. For example, those with cardiovascular disease, diabetes, and lifestyle factors such as cigarette smoking may be ruled out as candidates for a prostatectomy. In older men, surveillance—known also as expectant management—is often suggested. In cases where recurrence occurs, radiation may be considered.

The surgical option has been challenged in the past few years, as advances take place in radiation oncology laboratories. But for those patients whose prime concern is sexual potency, the scale so far seems to weigh heavily on the side of surgery. For younger men, diagnosed early with the disease, the pertinent question is, how does radical prostatectomy compare with other interventions such as pelvic radiation and brachytherapy?

For certain, surgery is associated with an immediate, precipitous loss of erectile function, which does not occur when radiation therapy is performed. It is, however, often recoverable when nerve sparing occurs. On the other hand, radiation therapy often results in a steady decline in erectile function as the body's cells are destroyed over time, within three to five years.

Dr. Burnett believes the next frontier in the clinical management of erectile dysfunction will focus on strategies that restore nerve function and find new ways to promote nerve growth. Research in these fields has already begun.

How to Read This Book

Most men do not talk among themselves about health issues, especially when it comes to prostate cancer. When a doctor tells them they have the disease, they can explode with fear. The air becomes saturated with terrifying questions: Why me? Am I going to die? How will the disease affect my life? What should I do? Where do I turn?

Given these circumstances, a man is apt to turn to his doctor for advice in making such judgments. That may be a starting point, but it is hardly the wise endgame. Studies show that doctors often offer suggestions based primarily on medical considerations, often ignoring the patient's lifestyle. All too often we hear of doctors advising patients to follow the course of treatment they are most familiar with instead of relating other treatments that may be more appropriate to the patient or, in some instances, that no treatment is appropriate. That being the case, a man can be expected to turn to his wife, girlfriend, partner, or good friend to assist in the research process, to help assess whether a second opinion may be needed in reaching a decision. The interviews presented here illustrate the importance of supporting the patient. They also demonstrate how encouragement can promote the healing process and bring about closer relationships among couples.

Doctors usually tell patients to read a good medical text to familiarize themselves with prostate cancer. They often will point out specific chapters that pertain to a patient's particular condition. The patient is encouraged to talk to others who have gone through the same treatments. *This book is prepared as a companion piece, putting a human face on a medical text.* Here we offer first-person accounts of patients who have undergone different kinds of treatments, pointing out the experiences they have encountered. Each story is selected to reveal details a reader wants to know—the issues, problems, difficulties, and triumphs. What treatment works for one does not necessarily work for another, but the format allows a reader to carefully weigh the prospects for a successful outcome as it pertains to him.

The architecture of this book is designed to be flexible, with first-person interviews with prostate cancer survivors who tell their own stories frankly and honestly, sharing their fears and hopes. Dr. Burnett comments to clarify and explain. Reading the book from cover to cover can provide an overview of the many variations prostate cancer can take. It can also reveal how patients differ in their approaches to solving their treatment dilemmas and how some, when faced with the choice of longevity versus lifestyle, deal with this difficult option. Or, you may choose to read sections that pertain directly to you and your particular situation.

Stories are grouped into sections according to the issues these men have had to face. In part I, we focus on the diagnosis of prostate cancer and the ramifications of coming to terms with it. In part II, we examine the various options and treatments. In part III, we hear some warnings from the interviewees based on their experiences. In part IV, we examine the aftereffects of prostate cancer treatments. Finally, we look at scientific frontiers as researchers search for breakthroughs.

In the individual stories, patients reveal intimate details about their personal struggles fighting prostate cancer, how they decided on an appropriate treatment, and what were the consequences of their decisions. Prostate cancer does not discriminate; it strikes ordinary people and celebrities alike. In so doing, it bonds together all those whom it affects into what many call a "reluctant brotherhood." You will hear from members of the brotherhood who tell of their experiences and share their wisdom and missteps so that others may benefit.

Many of the cases offered include the viewpoints of wives and partners. While not every story has a rosy outcome, each one demonstrates a healthy outlook and a desire to survive and live life to the fullest. Communication between patients, wives, and partners is an essential ingredient in the decision-making process, as these interviews clearly show. At the same time, it allows those who are closest to the patient to understand the trauma he is undergoing and help promote better understanding among wives or partners and other members of the family.

Following each interviewee's story is a section titled "The Doctor's Notebook," which features Dr. Burnett's own analysis of the patient's situation along with other facts about prostate cancer. Dr. Burnett adds an expert's perspective on the medical and psychological considerations behind each patient's story. In several chapters, following "The Doctor's Notebook" is a section titled "Prescriptive Information," which offers additional facts, information, and treatment options. Taken together, the two parts of each chapter may be of particular interest to physicians and medical caretakers in supplying important feedback they might otherwise not be privy to. In disseminating such information, we hope to increase the understanding and sensitivities of those whose charge is to offer the best medical care possible to prostate cancer patients and their families.

Please note that the names of physicians referred to by patients in their personal accounts have been changed for protection of privacy. With the exception of references to my coauthor, Dr. Arthur L. Burnett II, and in instances where specific permission has been granted, the names of doctors I allude to are pseudonyms. Ages cited refer to the time the interviews took place.

PART I

Diagnosis and Coming to Terms

1

Your Life in Our Hands

Every week I see the harsh realities and uncertainties faced by many of my patients who require management for prostate cancer. In some respects, their dilemmas are my own because my involvement in their care means that I also anguish in wanting the very best outcomes for them. Many demands plague decisions for management of this disease, from contemplating the courses of current treatment options to reconciling potential risks. Our charge as clinical specialists in the field is to help patients with this onerous task, starting with providing basic guidance and information. Quite often, we are further called upon to deliver an unequivocal, self-assured directive in response to the innocent request, "Tell me what I should do now, doc." The frequent assumption is that physicians can always know the best answer and perhaps even predict an optimal outcome. But when it comes to prostate cancer, easy answers are not always available and the most favorable outcomes are not always possible. The fact is that to this day, prostate cancer remains a very challenging clinical management problem. That is true for the patient and his family and many times no less so for their dedicated doctors. This struggle continues despite many recent promising strides that have been made in the science and clinical practice surrounding this important disease.

In the past, prostate cancer was often trivialized, owing in part to inaccuracies and delays in its diagnosis as well as to the dearth of satisfactory treatments. And contributing to this earlier attitude was the notion that this disease represented an affliction only of older men who would likely die from other medical causes. However, in the twenty-first century, as other serious health conditions such as heart disease and diabetes have become better addressed, and consequently as life expectancy has steadily increased, prostate cancer is no longer looked upon as a problem of older men with little lifetime consequences. Today, we are witnessing a heightened public awareness of the threat posed by prostate cancer, and for good reason.

The reality is that prostate cancer is now the leading solid-organ malignancy in men in the United States, second only to lung cancer as a cause of cancer-related deaths. The good news is that two major weapons have arrived to confront prostate cancer: better diagnostic tools and improved approaches for effective treatment. For example, the advent of prostate-specific antigen (PSA) testing has facilitated early diagnosis, and other diagnostic techniques such as prostate cancer imaging and prostate biopsy methodology have been further developed to improve assessments of cancer progression and risk of death. Refinements in treatment, ranging across domains of surgery and radiation therapy, have also translated into better cancer control with reduced side effects.

Still, in the ongoing war against prostate cancer, some challenges persist, while new ones have arisen. An ongoing controversy, for instance, is whether the need exists for treatment of *all* presentations of the disease. In other words, should every patient whose tests reveal some presence of cancer cells be up for medical treatment? Or does the case call merely for supervised observation? The core issue here is whether early-stage, low-profile presentations of the disease, which are highly treatable, actually warrant treatment. The fact of the matter is that some patients may indeed die from a non–prostate cancer illness while harboring latent prostate cancer with little likelihood of progression and no bearing on their health performance and life expectancy. So the charge at hand is to discern who is at risk of dying from the disease and definitely needs treatment, and who is not at such risk and can be managed with expectant monitoring. We doctors often refer to this close surveillance technique as watchful waiting, following expectantly, or the newer term, expectant management. This challenge persists in many respects, despite the increasing availability of supposedly predictive diagnostic instruments, nomograms, algorithms, and so forth.

Dilemmas also revolve around determining which treatment is most appropriate for specific presentations of the disease. This concern is particularly relevant for prostate cancer that is clinically localized (confined to the prostate and not spread throughout the body). Here, the issue is that there are multiple treatment options from which to choose. Far from an easy decision, it can become a complicated matter made more challenging lately in light of the emergence of various new, but not proven to be better, treatment approaches. These include laparoscopic and robotic surgeries in the domain of surgery and interstitial seeds (brachytherapy) in the domain of radiation treatments. In my opinion, best choices do exist in certain situations, such as radical prostatectomy to achieve definitive disease eradication for the relatively young man with early-stage disease and a very good life expectancy (greater than ten years). Unfortunately, the best choices often remain hotly debated because data remain lacking at this time, and we do not know unequivocally which treatment alternative offers superior cancer control outcomes. In the same way, because accurate data are currently limited with respect to sexual, urinary, and bowel function side effects resulting from various treatments, arguments for broadly superior functional recovery outcomes with any select treatment cannot be substantiated. This dilemma has become increasingly important today, as more and more attention is given to intervening early while maintaining quality of life objectives.

The prostate cancer surgeon, as much as any other specialist in various disciplines applied in the clinical management of this disease, must confront and resolve these ongoing realities for the interest of our patients. In practice, we aim to counsel our patients wisely and assist them in making the very best decision regarding their management. Our responsibility is to inform them truthfully and completely about the procedures, risks, and expectations associated with all therapeutic options. To the best of our ability, even when answers are not completely known, we need to help patients with the most accurate information possible in all areas, including issues of cancer control and functional recovery outcomes associated with various treatments. It is a shared responsibility that weighs heavily upon me.

Commonly enough, we encounter clinical predicaments that are beyond our ability to control. For instance, I have seen rather young patients with supposedly long lives still to live—say, men in their forties or early fifties—who have been dealt the plight of highly aggressive or advanced prostate cancers and are hopeful that I may be able to cure their disease. These situations are very tough to handle because of the regrettable truth that surgery will not be successful in achieving disease eradication. Supporting these patients requires that I summon an inner strength, a resolve about the matter: that these patients may have a treatable but not curable disease and that I am unable to bring them a cure. In fact, as a surgeon, one has to accept situations in which surgery is not useful because it would likely fail to be curative even despite a heroic attempt. I have learned that while it is important to be secure about oneself, it is also appropriate not to have an over-estimation of one's ability. Yet along the way it is important to remain positive and encouraging while conveying the truth about difficult situations.

Of course, the performance of these duties would be expected for any health-care professional acting within his or her specialty domain. I mention this role only to emphasize the absolute commitment we specialists must possess for our patients in light of our professional calling. In my view, it is particularly important for surgeons, who regularly hold someone's precious life literally in our hands when we go about applying the craft of surgery, and may with every precise—or imprecise—surgical maneuver change a bodily function or way of life.

Introspectively, I feel privileged and humbled amid these pro-fessional tests of character. I believe I have been gifted with talents, both mentally and physically, to do what I do as a surgeon, and I feel that putting them to use at the very highest level fulfills this gift. A further privilege is the trust placed in us by our patients, almost as if it were to be automatically bestowed because of an official rank. I view this regard as a special honor, which I must earn with the care of every patient. My promise to my patients, as a condition of this relationship, is that I serve them always, particularly in difficult times.

My philosophy in patient care is to devote myself completely to the individual patient. This self-awareness echoes the quote credited to the eminent Harvard-trained physician Dr. Francis Weld Peabody, who espoused that "the secret of the care of the patient is in caring for the patient." Caring for grateful patients can be a strong motivational force for practitioners of medicine, since it offers a reward perhaps greater than any other: purposefully affecting someone else's life. The fulfillment I gain by my actions as one human being administering to another is essentially that of knowing I was able to make a positive difference for somebody else.

I am delighted to have had the opportunity to partner with Norman Morris in the creation of this book. I know how important it has been for him to provide a resource for others finding themselves diagnosed with prostate cancer and then grappling with its many realities and uncertainties. I consider it his triumph to have put together his testimony as a prostate cancer survivor as well as the inspirational stories of other patients into a lasting written form that may help others. My many conversations with Norman have been most instructive. He related to me his observation that meager information exists in published form regarding personal experiences with the disease, although many books are available to report on the facts of the disease. The stories of the interviewees in this book reflect the resilience and frequently upbeat human spirit of patients who march on in the face of life's misdeeds and imperfections, including the unfairness of their disease and even the shortcomings of the medical field. It is hoped that in sharing them honestly, knowing that not all tell spectacular outcomes, this book fills a void. Norman also furthered my appreciation of the doctor-patient relationship, conveying the emotional value of a strong, genuine interaction. I have also appreciated from him that the prostate cancer surgeon can play a much more substantial role than just being a technician who skillfully removes prostate glands. Rather, the vocation includes that of counselor, advocate, and fellow human being.

Prescriptive Information

Basic Facts about Prostate Cancer

When it comes to matters of health, the vast majority of men prefer dealing with them on a need-to-know basis. Take the prostate, for example. It's not exactly a hot topic in the locker room. Show me the man who knows he even has a prostate or knows anything about it—or even mentions the word—and I'll show you a man who has met his prostate because it has caused him a problem. What kind of problem? Well, maybe he's running to the bathroom a lot. Maybe he's developed a burning sensation when he urinates. He could have a benign problem called prostatitis, a bacterial infection that a trip to the doctor could take care of with an antibiotic. Or maybe he's seen those TV ads that talk about an enlarged prostate. Could that be causing his problem? Maybe. Maybe not.

It's enough to confound a man and even drive him to a urologist. He may be worrying that whatever is bothering him is laying the groundwork for prostate cancer. The idea that prostatitis or an enlarged prostate (known as benign prostatic hyperplasia, or BPH) will inevitably lead to cancer is not true. And in the minds of many people, the real facts about prostatitis, BPH, and prostate cancer—the three major problems that the prostate can cause—are so often unclear, fuzzy, or downright wrong that it's important to have a good understanding about the prostate, what it does and what it does not do, and how you can learn to deal with any issues it may cause. Below we will present the facts and separate them from the misconceptions that are so prevalent.

Lifting the Fog of Confusion over Prostate Cancer

The fog that hangs over everything about prostate cancer is thick and hazardous for travelers. Those who must maneuver through it can easily become confused and not know which roads to take or where they will lead. That goes for *awareness*—recognizing there could be dangers ahead. It goes for *detection*—looking for signs of danger. It goes for early *diagnosis*—deciding whether to proceed or keep your foot lightly on the brake pedal. It goes for *treatment*—knowing how and where to steer if a hazard is spotted. And finally, it goes for the *management of late disease or functional setbacks*. We must find the ways to proceed safely by slipping through this miasma. It is not always easy, but with prudence, research, and good judgment we can do it and minimize the risky elements of chance or luck.

Awareness

Thanks to all of those pharmaceutical ads on television promoting prostate health, many men are becoming more aware that they have this thing called a prostate. They may know little about this gland until one day maybe they have some difficulty urinating or they find themselves running to the bathroom frequently. The commercials generally talk about BPH or an enlargement of the prostate. And they suggest that to be sure the condition *is* benign, only your doctor can tell. The truth is, only your doctor can tell if you are suffering from an enlarged prostate that causes urinary discomfort, if you have prostatitis, an inflammation of the prostate gland, or *if you have prostate cancer*! The weird thing, though, is that prostate cancer may not be accompanied by pain or by any other recognizable symptom. So how do you know?

What you must understand is that an overwhelming majority of men at some time in their lives will be affected by prostate problems. Some of these problems will be benign, and some will be cancerous. The prostate gland plays a role in reproduction, but oddly enough, it is not essential for that task. It is more of an aid in the process. Its main job apparently is to safeguard the reproductive tract from an infection in the urinary tract. So it is not a vital organ. Yet it is remarkable how such a small gland can cause such incredible confusion with potential consequences. And because prostate cancer can move like a silent intruder, lurking about and causing no symptoms, it is critical that men become aware that one day trouble can be brewing and the intruder may make his move. Awareness is the first weapon in the arsenal of defending against prostate cancer.

Detection

The American Cancer Society (ACS) estimated that new cases of prostate cancer in the United States by year's end in 2009 would reach about 192,000. That is somewhat more than in 2008 but less than in years gone by; still, prostate cancer remains the most frequently diagnosed cancer in men. For reasons that remain unclear, the incidence rates among African American men are significantly higher than among the white population. Incidence rates in general are substantially higher than they were over the last twenty years, reflecting increased screening for prostate cancer with the PSA blood test, especially among younger men.

Although death rates have been declining among white and African American men since the 1990s, the rates in the African American community remain more than twice as high as those of white men. In fact, it is estimated that in 2007 the African American death rate for prostate cancer was 2.4 times higher! Studies suggest that socioeconomic factors lie at the heart of the disparities, influencing the entire spectrum of cancer from prevention and early detection to treatment, quality of life, and survival. ACS figures show that compared with 10 percent of the white population, 24 percent of African Americans live below the poverty line. Moreover, 20 percent of African Americans are underinsured, while only 11 percent of white Americans lack health insurance. The result is that the poor and uninsured are subjected to poor diets, lack of sufficient physical activity, and lack of access to screening tests and appropriate follow-up. They are also more likely to be treated for prostate cancer at late stages of the disease, to receive substandard clinical care and services, and to die from their cancers. If awareness, then, is the first weapon in the arsenal to deal with a possible incursion of prostate cancer, the second and more powerful one is detection.

Up until the 1980s the principal means of trying to determine if a man had prostate cancer was the digital rectal exam (DRE). Then along came a newer tool, the PSA, a simple blood test meant to provide a better means of identifying prostate cancer. If the test suggested the possible presence of cancer cells, the follow-up was a biopsy to confirm the suspicion. Clinical studies showed that about a third of the men with a PSA over 4 had a localized prostate cancer upon biopsy. By the early 1990s, PSA testing was gaining in popularity.

Widespread screening set off a national debate over the question of whether early PSA testing saves lives. In the March 2009 issue of the *New England Journal of Medicine*, two studies addressed the question, but they appeared to contradict each other. A landmark European project involving seven countries and 162,000 men who were followed for as long as fourteen years concluded that PSA testing *can* save lives (there was a 27 percent decrease in prostate cancer deaths). In contrast, a U.S. project, half as large, over seven years, *showed no improvement in deaths* from prostate cancer. Which is right and what should you believe? How should a man decide if and when to get tested?

Dr. Burnett says there are some problems in the European studies, but he agrees with Johns Hopkins's Distinguished Service Professor of Urology, Patrick C. Walsh, that there are deep flaws in the U.S. project and that longer-range studies are needed. Nonetheless, Dr. Walsh believes the European scientists are on the right track and that PSA testing can reduce deaths from prostate cancer.

So the answer to the question "Should I get tested?" is this: the best advice experts agree on is that men should consult with their physicians, and that physicians in turn must make sure that patients are given information about the benefits and limitations of testing, so they can make informed decisions about whether to be tested or not. Generally speaking, if you are between the ages of fifty-five and sixty-nine and in good health and want to avoid prostate cancer, you may want to consider being tested. If you are in a high-risk group you should definitely consider being tested. If you are African American, you may want to think about being tested at about age forty. In any case, you will always want to consult with your physician.

There is a lot of prostate cancer out there that may be of low threat, and patients should know that the PSA test is an imperfect tool, although it is the best we have so far. Low-threat disease is prevalent in many men as they age, and it does not necessarily mean it will become an issue in their lifetime. Those men need not necessarily be treated. The PSA test in and of itself does not pose a threat. When we speak of "threat," what is implied is what could follow—namely, a biopsy and treatments. Biopsies could cause issues for some patients, such as discomfort, bleeding, and rarely infection. Treatments pose the issues of incontinence and sexual dysfunction. So PSA testing carries with it the implication that the test could potentially lead to biopsy and treatment. Overly aggressive treatment, when not necessary to save a man's life, is the real issue. At a time when the country is concerned with controlling the huge cost of national health care, the dilemma of overtreatment or unnecessary treatment is being scrutinized. Again, it is the physician's responsibility to point to the risks associated with testing and treatment, if appropriate, as well as the risks of not testing and missing an opportunity for treatment, and to encourage men who would likely benefit from treatment to get it.

Treatment

Over the past several decades, research scientists and urologists have made unimaginable strides in the diagnosis and treatment of prostate diseases. New therapies and innovative techniques have saved thousands of lives. In the treatment of BPH, for instance, the application of new therapies for shrinking the prostate has reduced the need for surgery. Doctors are now able to better understand the underlying causes of prostatitis (a benign condition) and treat the inflammation or infection successfully. Nevertheless, men who are confronted with these prostate problems have every right to wonder: Is my condition serious? Am I okay? If I do have BPH, should I take medicine or go for surgery? If I think I'm getting symptoms of prostatitis, should I take an antibiotic? Am I being confronted with prostate cancer? Supposing I do have prostate cancer, is it life-threatening? When it comes to matters concerning the prostate, one size does not fit all. Prostate diseases are complex and variable. What works for your friend may not work for you. Besides, knowledge of prostate cancer keeps growing. But the tough part is that myths and misconceptions abound, so how do you sort them out from good authoritative information? We hope that this book will help you learn how others have grappled with these questions and how they have attempted to find the answers to their individual issues.

Major Treatment Choices for Prostate Cancer

The prostate cancer patient must see himself as the ultimate decision maker in choosing the treatment he will opt for. The doctor may try to help, as may family members or friends, but in the end the patient must make the final choice. Sorting through these options can be confusing and often they are not easily understood. The patient must ask the doctor questions. A lot of questions. There are the outcomes to consider. To some, lifestyle may outweigh longevity. To others, the potential for a cure may far outweigh the potential consequences of lengthy incontinence or impotence.

These can be hard choices. And they belong to the patient who must make them. The patient must also be certain to ask the doctor how many times he or she has performed a particular therapy. It is imperative to make a judgment about the doctor's skill and experience and to determine a level of comfort with the doctor's manner. In later chapters, you can get the details on various treatments. But for now we would like to take you on a brief journey to give you a grasp of the concepts underlying the major prostate cancer treatments. Fasten your seat belt.

Let's think about treatments as a navigational system (GPS) in a car. The GPS determines the location of your car using satellites that orbit overhead and pinpoint where you are. When you set it, the GPS knows its destination and follows a route to get there.

The GPS is very accurate in following clearly marked roads. But sadly, as it gets into rural or less densely populated areas where roads are not clearly marked—rustic dirt roads, for example—it becomes less precise and can falter. You may have to do the old-fashioned thing: get out of your car and ask somebody how to find the address you're looking for.

Many have referred to the radical prostatectomy as the "gold standard" of therapies. Unfortunately, surgery is not always appropriate for everybody. But think of surgery in this instance as setting the destination (cancer-free; best outcomes). Hopefully, this GPS will take you down clearly marked roads straight to your destination with no confusion. The other two main therapies (external beam radiation and "seeds") set the GPS to the same cancer-free destination. But in each case, getting there can become a challenge for the system.

Newer and more interesting therapies are also coming along. Some show more promise than others. But the efficacy of many of these new therapies is uncertain because no long-term studies are yet available. How close they will bring you to your destination is yet unclear.

If the cancer is very advanced, your treatments may become more difficult and your path may become more elusive. You may not quite get to your destination, but the chances that you will get very close get better as advances in research continue.

In sum, as progress in differing treatment may areas improves and continues to advance, the chances of getting where you want to go—cancer-free and able to live life to the fullest—become greater and less elusive.

2

Norman S. Morris
The End of an Odyssey

I remember the first time I experienced the pain—the intense, screaming bladder, on fire, and the crushing pressure that broke right through my sound sleep, hurling me like a pitched ball straight down the hall to our bathroom. I remember the effort to urinate to relieve the pressure and the insistent feeling of fire. And the pythonlike pressure around my bladder that would not surrender. I could hardly wait for daybreak to see the urologist.

Dr. Jacob Lax found some blood in my urine and prescribed an antibiotic, and after one capsule the pain began to ease; within a few more hours, and a second capsule, it was miraculously and completely gone. The doctor called the condition prostatitis, an inflammation of the prostate gland, and it became a new catchword in my vocabulary. That's when I discovered that this little prostate of mine was pretty vital to my existence. The prostate, about the size of a walnut or a large strawberry, has been described by some as being the equivalent of Grand Central Station, meaning connections to the male reproductive and urinary systems, rectum, major arteries, and delicate nerve bundles run, like tracks, in and around it. Any disruption to that "station" can affect service in the rest of the body, as any New York City commuter can understand.

Within the prostate and arriving on track one is the urethra, a tube that carries urine from the bladder out of the body. Dr. Lax's first step was to perform a digital rectal exam (DRE). The back wall of the prostate lies flat up against the rectal wall, so the doctor reaches in to see if he can feel any lumps on the prostate wall. They are hard like knuckles. Those lumps are not necessarily cancerous. But they may be regarded by the physician as "suspects" or "nodules of interest."

Dr. Lax found some of these suspicious fellows and went to step two. He drew a blood sample and sent it off to a lab for the PSA test; the results came back an auspicious 1.2. So what did that mean?

PSA (prostate-specific antigen) is an enzyme that the prostate releases into the bloodstream. Elevated levels of the enzyme *can* signal prostate cancer. I emphasize the word "can" here because, as the old song goes, "it ain't necessarily so." While cancer may elevate the level of PSA, so may other factors. The mystery then is left to the doctor to solve, and his level of expertise becomes one of vital concern. Does this patient have cancer?

There was blood in my urine, but all indications were that my urinary incursions were purely bacteriological. My bouts with prostatitis would strike on average every six months over a stretch of some ten years. My case was turning into an enigma, because over those ten years my DRE seemed to Dr. Lax to remain unchanged. "About the same," he kept reiterating. "A little hardness on the right lobe of the prostate." This indicated possible minimal prostate cancer, but at the same time I had a PSA of only 1.2, indicating probably no cancer, certainly little or nothing to be concerned about.

Some urological cases are more easily diagnosed than others, particularly when it comes to prostatitis. That my PSA remained steady and low-grade mystified Dr. Lax; still, he felt there was no need to do a biopsy and no real need for concern. He told me he didn't want to play havoc with my quality of life. My wife and I were both Dr. Lax's patients. Not only did we share the same doctor, but we even took the same antibiotic medications. She was suffering from chronic cystitis and I from prostatitis. We were a urologist's dream.

As time passed, however, Dr. Lax became more and more disturbed by the persistent recurrence of my bacteriological infections and by the contraindications. He finally brought my case before an assembled group of colleagues at a urological seminar. "To a man," he told me afterward, "they advocated a policy of wait and see." And so we did just that. Until one particularly painful prostatitis flare-up.

Dr. Lax sat me down in his office and told me how distressed he had become. The PSA remained steady at 1.2, but he thought he now felt a little more hardness on the prostate wall. I can tell you that you do not want to see distress registered on your urologist's face. But there it was. Dr. Lax said emphatically that the waiting time was over. The time to do a biopsy had arrived.

His procedure called for snipping eight core samples of prostate tissue. Somebody who had likened the prostate to a strawberry said the cores were no bigger than the tiny black seeds on top. Removing each one amounted to nothing more and nothing less than a tiny pinch. That feeling can hardly be compared to the body blow that came next with the news that *one* of those eight strawberry seeds was cancerous!

Pathologists, though, reported only a moderate Gleason score of 6. (The Gleason score is a way of classifying the severity of cancer based on how it looks under a microscope.) A great deal of time had been consumed with the wait-and-see course. Nearly twelve years! Granted, the conflicting signals produced no red flags for our urologist, only a complicated riddle of *CSI* proportions. But clearly my family's concern rang out for a second opinion.

My own thoughts, I recall, became muddled, confused, unaccepting. If I was experiencing shock, I would have to say that it became muted, and I began slipping into denial. But I am not psychologically ever willing to remain in that frame of mind. I have trained myself to get a grip on tough situations. What happened next was the realization that I had to solve this problem. I couldn't afford to wallow. I had to move ahead and make decisions.

Finding the medical expert—whether a surgeon or a radiation oncologist—to render that second opinion can become a demanding preoccupation, one entailing thorough research and reaching out to trusted physicians, family members, and friends who may have firsthand experience and/or knowledge of the disease and different treatments. In any event, one admonition must be kept in mind: the chosen practitioner should always be measured by experience and proficiency in carrying out the treatment or course of action. Perhaps a good rule of thumb, I learned, is to exclude any doctor who performs less than a hundred procedures a year!

My choice for the second opinion was the Brady Urological Institute at Johns Hopkins in Baltimore, and I wasted little time making an appointment with one of the hospital's foremost surgeons, Dr. Arthur Burnett. Dr. Burnett is a man whose very presence exudes warmth and confidence without the slightest trace of medical hubris. His rare empathy and sensibility are so apparent that he is able almost immediately to allay a patient's anxieties.

After methodically reviewing my medical records and charts, Dr. Burnett slipped on a pair of the famous Hopkins purple exam gloves and went straight to the business of performing the DRE. Moments later came *his* report: the prostate wall felt hard as concrete. Before I knew it, I found myself downstairs at the lab. And when the results came back a few days later, along with the pathology report, Dr. Burnett's predictions were confirmed, right on the mark: a PSA of 4, not 1.2, as reported by the New Jersey pathologists, and a Gleason score of 8, not 6, as suggested by the same pathology group.

I listened intently when Dr. Burnett told me he was certain that if I were to continue the course of wait and see, I could certainly live comfortably for another three years. Those words snapped me to attention. With surgery, he went on, I could add fifteen, perhaps twenty years. His concern, however, was that Dr. Lax had waited too long for a biopsy—that the window of opportunity for good outcomes might already have closed. The gravity of his words terrified me and my wife. The decision—which way to go—would be mine and mine alone. Which door revealed the lady and which door the tiger?

Dr. Burnett handed me a book titled *Dr. Patrick Walsh's Guide to Surviving Prostate Cancer*. I read enough about the radical prostatectomy to convince myself that surgery represented the gold standard of therapies. There were other options, like seed implants and external beam therapies and hormone treatments, each with promised benefits, yet each with downsides unacceptable to me. I reasoned that surgery came closest to my goals, which were first and foremost survival and elimination of the cancer, and second, the best prospects for quality of life. I put the Walsh book down before I got to the part that talked about possible postsurgical outcomes. I had had enough. I was ready to act. Who knew that there were other doors concealing critters other than a tiger and a lady? Not me!

A great deal of preparation is required before a patient undergoes a radical prostatectomy. The Johns Hopkins instructions called for a physical exam by my internist. Next came an EKG provided by my cardiologist, then a donation of three pints of the patient's own blood for possible transfusion during and after the operation. This kind of self–blood donation is called autologous transfusion, and the idea is to avoid any possibility that you receive someone else's blood contaminated with HIV or hepatitis.

All bureaucracies can take a lesson from Johns Hopkins, where administrative systems work with the efficiency of a quartz timepiece. I saw that from the minute I checked in to the minute I checked out. The key to it all is Hopkins's famous computerized orange plastic card that allows every staff member and caregiver to protect your identity and track your medical conditions and medications. It speeds you along, tears down language barriers, and helps avoid mistakes.

My medical journey began on the morning of March 20, 2002. I had a choice of anesthesia—general or spinal. I chose general. I really had no desire to watch the proceedings. It was cold in the operating room. I remember that. One of the nurses saw me shivering and came over to cover me with a warm blanket. God, did that feel good. I began to feel warm all over. Another nurse approached, smiled, and whispered, "It's always cold in here, but we'll keep you warm." Moments later I saw Dr. Burnett arrive in a blue surgical gown, along with the team of assisting physicians. He came over and said, "Hi, Mr. Morris, how you doing?" He was smiling. He is always smiling. "Looking good in that nightcap." I don't remember much more. I was beginning to feel very, very sleepy. Very, very . . . and then . . .

I woke up. "It's all over," a nurse said. "You did just great. They're going to take you down to recovery now. And Dr. Burnett will be calling your wife and she'll meet you down there."

What you lose in a prostatectomy is not only your rogue gland but also your modesty. One patient I spoke with in the hospital put it this way: "There are doctors and nurses, as well as residents, interns, medical students, and aides of both sexes and sundry ages, who will be checking you and your bodily functions every few hours. They will not only be viewing and discussing, but also probing and handling your heretofore private parts that are now misshapen and traumatized from the surgery."

When I left the recovery area, aides carefully lifted me onto a gurney and began wheeling me down a maze of corridors. I was still groggy from the anesthesia and my eyes began following the endless rows of fluorescent ceiling fixtures as we moved along through double doors that opened like magic. When we reached my room, nurses appeared as the aides gently helped me shift from the gurney onto the bed and then disappeared down the hall.

The nurses quickly transferred the IV from the gurney to the room unit, hooked me up to a heart monitor, and began periodically checking my blood pressure. The one annoyance I found was the thigh-high open-toed stockings you are required to wear to prevent blood clots. I hated the feeling of these stockings. They were not my thing. After a while a nurse wrapped my calves in cuffs that automatically inflated and deflated—another device to prevent clotting by encouraging the blood to flow freely in my legs.

Toward the end of the day, Dr. Burnett came to my bedside, speaking the words I had been waiting, with all my fingers crossed, to hear. "I am confident," he said, "we got all the cancer." You cannot imagine my euphoria, my complete, unfettered sense of relief! "The cancer was aggressive," he continued, "but pretty much confined to the capsule. The only thing was that some of it got over the right side and we had to take the bundle. The good news is that you're cancer-free."

I was too elated over the major news to pay much attention to that business about his having to remove "the bundle." For all I knew, he could have been talking about the laundry. The lesson I was to learn was that I should have finished the second part of the Walsh book, the part that talks about bundles and post-operative outcomes.

As soon as my vitals looked good and stable, the nurses introduced me to the Foley catheter. During the operation, while the many "tracks" are rerouted, the Foley catheter is inserted in the penis, threaded through it, and attached to the bladder. My nurse explained that the urine then collects in a plastic bag taped to my leg. She patiently showed me how to empty the bag. As you might imagine, patients concur it may well be the most disagreeable part of the prostatectomy. On average, the patient will be toting the Foley catheter around for about fourteen days like some sort of ball and chain.

The day after surgery, I was out of bed and my nurse removed the urine collection bag and suspended it from an IV trolley. She gently took me by the arm and accompanied me on my first post-op walk down the corridor. Those first steps were encouraging but at the same time exhausting. We repeated that exercise on the following days, gradually increasing the walking distance and pace until I felt strong enough to walk unassisted, toting the IV trolley with more and more ease.

My hospital stay amounted to three days, during which time I was primed to make certain that all systems were A-okay: lungs, heart, no blood clotting threats, and all the rest. Doctors assured me that the swelling of my scrotum was perfectly normal and that it would disappear in a few days. They pronounced me to be in great shape and I was released to return home.

A return to normal activity after a radical prostatectomy generally can take from six to eight weeks. The PSA level can't be expected to drop dramatically until four to five weeks have gone by. All radical prostatectomy patients will endure degrees of urinary incontinence following surgery. The amount of time required to become dry varies widely. For the fortunate few it can be only a matter of days. For others it can take weeks, months, or longer. Older men can be troubled with it for years. All patients are urged to practice Kegel exercises that strengthen the pelvic muscles and help end urinary incontinence.

Many stories end here. Some, like mine, do not. Bear in mind that all human bodies are different. Even the best identically performed procedures don't guarantee identical results. There's no telling how our cells will react to being stretched and pulled or cut or radiated during whatever treatment the best doctors perform. We go by statistics, risks, and chances—and, of course, hopes. Medicine, after all, is as much an art as it is a science.

One evening in early July 2002, about four months after my discharge from Johns Hopkins, as I was getting ready for bed, my wife noticed that my right leg had suddenly ballooned to *twice* the size of my left from the top of my thigh right down to my ankle. We were startled and concerned and immediately put in a call to Dr. Burnett.

The next morning we were back in Baltimore and Dr. Burnett was taking a look at this unexpected edema. He explained that in the off chance that edema (swelling) occurs, it happens immediately after the operation, but this was four months later. He was convinced that for lymphatic fluid to back up like this was a most unusual occurrence and the first thing to try was inserting a drain. It would be done by another surgeon specializing in this kind of trauma.

The drain was inserted during an overnight stay at Hopkins, and then we felt secure enough to undertake a vacation we had planned to Cape Cod. The Foley catheter was long gone, but I once again had a plastic bag (drain) taped to my leg, well hidden under sweatpants or baggy shorts. After two days or so on the cape, I developed a high fever. It became all too apparent that the drain had somehow become infected. I had no choice but to return to Baltimore, this time to remove the drain. The edema had not disappeared and getting rid of it seemed to be eluding doctors.

It did not, however, seem to elude my internist in West Orange, New Jersey, Dr. Jim Maguire. He had a suggestion: buy some antiembolism stockings, the ones I hated so much, the kind they use after surgery to prevent clots. I thought he was "reaching," and that nothing could possibly come of it. The very idea of wearing these stockings for an indeterminate period of time struck me as uncomfortable and unlikely to help. I was beside myself to find stockings with closed toes, and when I did, I began wearing them every day with little hope that they would accomplish anything. But I would play out this string.

In August, I began to believe I was turning into a professional patient. The prostatectomy was behind me. I was dealing with the edema issue. But there I was, back in Dr. Maguire's office with a new problem, and we hadn't even completely worked out the edema issue. As I sat and told him about a new gripping pain I was experiencing in my abdomen, I was sure Dr. Maguire thought I was some sort of neurotic. I felt ashamed to present another problem for him to solve, but I had little choice because sometimes the pain had me doubled over. I climbed up on his examining table and it didn't take him long to come to a conclusion. "Well, you've got a large groin hernia. You need to see a surgeon."

That would make three operations in five months! And it presented a bigger problem. We had booked a trip to Italy long ago. It had taken a lot of time and research, and all our plans were made. Besides, we were traveling with another couple. I just could not face the possibility that this surgery would kill the trip. Certainly, there would be no way I could travel with the hernia. And I could not understand the origin of a hernia. Dr. Burnett later explained that the hernia was not at the surgical incision site. It was in the groin. The prostatectomy did not involve any sort of direct dissection or manipulation of the groin, but following surgical closure of the wound the groin area became susceptible to some "give." As a man ages, Dr. Burnett explains, already weakened structures in the abdominal region can allow a hernia to develop.

The hernia operation would take place near where we lived in New Jersey. My newest surgeon assured me that I didn't have to cancel our travel plans. He performed the operation a week after the consultation, and after three weeks' time, unbelievably, I was back on my feet, minus a hernia and feeling well enough to travel.

My wife, meanwhile, who has been the constant mainstay of my life, suddenly crashed into a psychological wall. She had been bearing the brunt of my seemingly endless physical problems and felt her resilience crumbling. She began sliding into a deep depression.

The thought of or mere allusion to our trip set her off. All she said she felt prepared to do was to sit in a corner and suck her thumb or climb into bed and pull the covers over her head. But I felt strongly that a trip to Italy was precisely what she needed, and along with her close friends urged her to get help. Her doctor felt that her issues were treatable with antidepression medication and agreed that a trip abroad would be the best part of the prescription.

I knew she was doing the best she could when she quietly joined in packing our bags. We made sure that one of those bags was filled with pads to deal with the urinary incontinence. That had not leveled off, and yet I had no intention of allowing it to get in our way.

We left for Italy in late September. The country, as so many people know, is a land of mountains and hills and endless stairways. And nothing could deter me from climbing hills and walking for stretches of miles. Urinary incontinence be damned. All throughout our travels I diligently wore my knee-high stockings except on the beach. And by the time we returned from Europe, something miraculous had happened. The edema had gradually dissipated, despite all the travel, up and down hills and mountains and stairways. Hats off to Dr. Jim Maguire. The pressure from the stockings had squeezed the lymphatic fluid right out of my leg, and there it was, back to normal size!

That was progress. But my story did not end there. Kegel exercises seemed to be slowing down the urinary incontinence. The number of pads I needed had been decreasing. Then suddenly one day the flow began *increasing*. I found myself resorting to as many as ten pads a day! Something terribly wrong was taking place! I was back to Baltimore in a New York minute toting a bag of heavy pads.

Could it be a sudden rupture around the neck of the bladder that was causing the problem? Dr. Burnett considered the possibility. He would first try the simplest of solutions and work his way through the problem. The first step was to inject what essentially was a plug of collagen to fill an interstitial opening.

The incontinence flow began to slow. I returned home to observe the results. The incontinence definitely improved—for several weeks. But then the levee broke again. The collagen had shifted. We tried again. More collagen. Another rupture. In all, over the next several months we had tried three injections of collagen, and none of the material was holding. On the last try, Dr. Burnett had his eureka moment. He recalled that the incontinence had dramatically worsened after catheterization associated with my hernia surgery. That event, he discovered, had affected the delicately reconstructed connection between the bladder neck and the urethra. In other words, a rupture had occurred at the point where the bladder neck and the urethra were joined. The medical description for this would be "disruption of the delicate anastomosis" (surgical union or connection). If you prefer, the simple word "tear" would suffice.

That is when Dr. Burnett produced the silver bullet: an artificial sphincter. It required yet another one-night stay in the hospital. This clever device has an inflatable cuff that encircles and squeezes the urethra and cuts off the flow of urine. To activate it, the user squeezes a pump, a valvelike bulb implanted in the scrotum, which causes the sterile fluid in the cuff to flow into a balloon. That action opens the cuff, permitting the urine to flow. The cuff stays open for approximately two minutes, allowing the patient to urinate, and then shuts off automatically, keeping the patient dry. If additional time is needed, no problem. The patient can repeat this simple routine.

Now, five years after installation of the artificial sphincter, I can happily report a most satisfactory outcome. Admittedly, I was one tough patient. But the bottom line is that I am alive and well! Free of cancer and finally free of those thick pads.

The Doctor's Notebook

Norman Morris has provided a lighthearted yet educational story about his confrontation with "the enemy," prostate cancer. It is most interesting as a surgeon to appreciate his story from the patient's perspective. Enlightening to me are several of his observations, particularly those on my behavior and comments. While stated with some dramatic effect, his remarks convey how the patient views what we surgeons say and do, especially as they struggle with a life-changing situation. It is clear that from the patient's perspective certain remarks about the confirmation of cancer, its risks, and how well a treatment fares are dramatically perceived.

Norman's story is illuminating in other ways as well. He reveals shortcomings associated with the diagnosis of prostate cancer in describing how difficult it may be for the doctor to make an early diagnosis. He had been under a urologist's watch and was considered to have prostatitis, inflammation of the prostate gland, a benign entity, but which may be symptomatic. The physician's attention can be directed toward relieving symptoms, thereby allaying the patient's distress.

The presence of prostatitis, though, can be a confounder for the diagnosis of prostate cancer. Prostatitis does not necessarily predict the presence of prostate cancer by our current level of understanding, and it does not necessarily direct surgeons to go about performing further invasive evaluation such as prostate biopsies. Sometimes it may cause elevations in the PSA; at other times it may change the texture of the prostate on digital rectal examination, making a diagnosis of prostate cancer problematic.

These circumstances could have been in play, affecting a more timely diagnosis of Norman's prostate cancer. It is interesting to note that his PSA value apparently did not rise much, which may occur with prostatitis. At the same time, his low PSA value (in the 0–4 range) persisted even with a prostate cancer diagnosis. A lesson here is that prostate cancer may occur with any PSA value, although a higher value would certainly lead to a greater degree of consternation. Again, all of these features reveal the challenges in making early prostate cancer diagnoses in many men.

Norman also highlights another very important matter in prostate cancer management. It is clear that he was prepared to take an active role in decision making regarding his treatment plan. He read up on the disease, considered his options, and made an intelligent decision about how he wanted to proceed. I consider this a tribute to him to have been such an active participant in his own health-care decisions. I believe all patients should follow his example.

Norman's story is punctuated by several apparent complications that followed surgery. He is telling the truth when he says that certain complications occur and patients should be prepared to know this. His account points to complications both common and uncommon.

Common are the complications of short-term urinary incontinence and erectile dysfunction. Indeed, urinary incontinence is observed in all men briefly following the surgery, with expectations that 95 percent will regain full urinary continence with no use of pads after several months. Erectile dysfunction also occurs in all men for at least a short period of time following surgery, with the expectation that the majority will recover their erections if they have undergone a "nerve-sparing" surgery and had preoperative potency. This recovery time is longer than that for urinary continence and may extend for as much as a year or two.

Remarkable for Norman is that his local extent of cancer was significant enough that he required a "non-nerve-sparing" prostatectomy that would certainly have affected his likelihood of erectile function recovery. In addition, the local extent of his disease influenced the surgical effects on his urinary sphincter, which probably in turn affected the extent of his urinary control recovery. These were potential risks that he was prepared to deal with based on our preoperative counseling and his desire to achieve complete eradication of the disease surgically, despite the possible expense of some loss of urinary and erectile functions. Another contributor to his loss of urinary control was that he had to face a hernia surgery within a few months of his radical prostatectomy. This apparently resulted from a traumatic urethral catheter placement after the hernia surgery that set him back with regard to his best urinary control recovery.

But Norman's story is important because it also shows that complications of radical prostatectomy can be managed. In his case, the urinary incontinence was initially managed with transurethral collagen injections, although ultimately he was best served by an artificial urinary sphincter. He reveals that the current management of his complications has been successful. And he maintains a happy existence primarily due to having had his highly aggressive and extensive prostate cancer cured. Norman also acknowledges the truth that other interventions for localized prostate cancer, including radiation, carry risks of sexual, urinary, and bowel function complications. Quite predictably, he would have faced similar complications had he sought radiation therapy as a treatment alternative.

Less common complications of surgery are featured in his testimony. He had developed a delayed presentation of a lymphocele. That is the collection of lymphatic fluid in the region of blood vessels coursing to the leg near the area of prostatic dissection. This complication can occur rarely when locations where lymph node tissue, removed at the time of prostatectomy, fails to stop draining, thus leading to fluid collection. It is a problem that can be handled with a minor surgical procedure in which a drain is placed through the skin to siphon off the accumulation of fluid. Afterward, his leg swelling resolved and the drain was simply removed. He also developed an inguinal (near the groin) hernia that can sometimes form after radical prostatectomy. This occasionally happens if a patient has weakened support structure in the inguinal region that becomes exposed after a radical prostatectomy. This problem also was corrected with appropriate action.

Despite this series of unusual difficulties, Norman has had a very successful outcome following his prostatectomy. His story reveals the potential for complications in association with radical prostatectomy, and more than likely the variety of his setbacks was greater than many other patients face. Yet his story is important in illustrating how potential complications can be overcome so that men can remain as functional as possible even after surgical prostate cancer treatment.

3

Richard Meyers

In the Race for Positive Outcomes, Lady Luck May Ride the Inside, but Better Preparation Can Carry the Day

Richard Meyers at sixty is the executive vice president of the First Trust Bank, a privately owned Philadelphia bank. As chief risk officer, he is the driving force behind his bank's business activities. His responsibilities include approving as much as 95 percent of all of the loan transactions it carries out. He and his wife, Donna, live in Wayne, Pennsylvania.

Despite his silver hair, Richard Meyers has a youthful face, along with brown eyes, an impressive mustache, and an easy smile. He's been a banker for thirty-eight years, the past nine with First Trust. Outside of his work, he has always spent a good deal of time participating in all manner of sports.

"Going back to my days in high school, I was an athlete. I went to Penn State and played basketball, baseball, and a lot of football. And softball, racquetball, and tennis. I still play tennis but not nearly as much as I used to. I've been a runner over the years, but the knees got a little sore, so I've given that up, but I do a lot of walking at this point. Today, I guess my primary activity is biking.

I've got a number of bikes at home, and every weekend, maybe one or two times a week, especially in the summertime, I take some fairly long rides. I actually take rides from Philadelphia to the Jersey shore and back; that's about a hundred and eighty miles over two days. I spend a lot of time on my bike, which gives me a good, vigorous, full exercise activity. And I'm very much into yoga and meditation for relaxation.

"Back in my forties, as part of my employment as a bank executive, I had a full physical every year. I wasn't thinking then about my prostate at all. I was more concerned about cholesterol and those kinds of things as opposed to the PSAs. The doctor was satisfied, so I was satisfied. The truth is I didn't know much at all about the prostate."

In his early fifties, Richard began dealing with some urinary infections. At about the same time, he was experiencing some sexual dysfunction, so he went to see a urologist to check things out. His doctor gave him some antibiotics and the infection cleared right up. "In talking to my physician I discovered it wasn't unusual for somebody my age to experience some slight sexual dysfunction. So I didn't take any medications. I didn't go on Viagra or anything. And the problem just seemed to disappear over time and never occurred again. No problem.

"Everything seemed absolutely normal. My PSA hadn't changed. It remained essentially 2.8—normal. But about three years later, I went and had another physical, and this time my PSA had jumped to 4.2! That didn't mean anything to me at the time. But that fifty percent change was obviously a red flag for my doctor. He told me it was probably nothing but said the only way to be sure was to see a urologist."

The urologist, Dr. Silverstein, did the biopsy, and when the results came back he immediately called Richard into his office. "I was alone with Dr. Silverstein. If I thought it was going to be something of a problem, my wife would probably have been there with me. But I wasn't thinking that way at all. In fact, my wife was going down to a beach house with a niece to spend a few days, and she asked if she should come along with me and I'd told her, 'No, it's not necessary. I'm just going to meet with Dr. Silverstein. He's just going to tell me everything's cool, and

I should just be attentive to this thing and make sure I'm getting my PSAs and all that. Just go.' But Dr. Silverstein's words hit me like a brick." One of the biopsy cores showed cancerous cells. He confirmed the PSA was now 4.2 and the Gleason was 6. He didn't feel there was anything immediate that had to be done, because he'd only found the cancer in one core, and his take was that the cancer wasn't that significant. "I was scared as hell. The notion of somebody telling me that I had cancer. I was damned scared *that I was going to die*! After my initial shock, I went into a little bit of 'why *me*?' in my head. Who picked this for me to have this? And then I quickly realized that this was not going to be too productive. And I tried to have a dialogue with Dr. Silverstein about it. Okay, what do I do? What should I be thinking about? How would you guide me in terms of getting information? How do I make a decision about what to do?"

It was late in the day, and Richard called his wife to tell her the bad news. She offered to come right home, but he told her to remain where she was. First, he said, he wanted to begin finding out what information he could about the disease, and then the two of them would put their heads together and figure out what course of action to take.

Back in his office, Richard spent many hours on the Internet trying to digest as much as he could. He spent the next two weeks continuing to gather information, having discussions with professionals, and reaching out to people who had prostate episodes in order to understand their experiences. "I was fairly ignorant about the task I had begun to deal with, and as task-oriented as I am, I was saying to myself, 'Look, I gotta get the information. I gotta know what I'm dealing with here, so I can reach out to other resources, so I can better understand . . . so I can make an informed judgment.' I decided that within a thirty-day period I would really make a decision if I could and move forward quickly. I was damned scared. But I kept reminding myself that I'd better stop feeling sorry for myself and deal with the problem.

"I knew I would be faced with questions from my children and from my mother and I didn't want to tell them until I had a body of knowledge to answer the very simple questions they were going to ask. I wanted to be in a position to say, 'Here's what I have to do.' And I wanted to give them a reasonable timetable as to when I was going to make a decision, so they would be in a position to understand what was going to happen. Of course, I was very concerned for my wife. She's a pretty resourceful lady, and I knew I could count on her to be a good partner and to support me. I knew we could work together and make the decision together. And I knew at the end of the day she would defer to me to make the decision about what to do. I believed, and as it turned out, she supported me to the nth degree and in the end was a great partner.

"I was not willing to stake my life on the opinion of a single urologist. So, after all the research, my plan was to go for *three* sets of opinions. I went to three institutions to be examined: the University of Pennsylvania, Jefferson [Medical School], and Johns Hopkins. Each of these institutions had surgical groups *and* radiation oncology groups, so I saw both groups at each institution on the same days of my visits. I came to clearly understand the alternatives. And clearly the ones I focused on were surgery, external radiation, and seed implants.

"As it related to seeds, I'd read about the process. I talked to doctors and to someone who had it done out in Seattle. I considered how long these procedures had actually been done and the body of information that was available to understand what comfort I could have [in terms of outcomes]. I decided the seeds procedure was just too early [i.e., too new a procedure to evaluate the long-term results]. I just didn't feel comfortable. I strongly considered radiation. But I guess clearly the crowning thought for me, after all I read and everybody I talked to, and being fifty-five years old and in real good health, without any other kinds of problems— my medical friends urged me to have surgery. Because if it was them, they said, they would want the cancer eradicated and out of their bodies. And they thought surgery was the gold standard and had the most predictable outcomes, that you could be comfortable with. Ultimately, that was the conclusion I came to. That's what I needed to do."

Richard and his wife ranked the possible outcomes. "Job number one was to get rid of the cancer once and for all. If I was left with incontinence and sexual dysfunction, so be it. And if I was left with no incontinence and with sexual dysfunction, I could live with that too. Fine!

"I had the prostatectomy at Johns Hopkins in November 2001. The surgery was easy. The anesthesiologist knew I had an interest in wines, so he offered me a cocktail he said was the equivalent of ten glasses of wine, and he said it would hit me as though I had drunk them all at one time. And he was right. I looked up and saw the clock. It was eight minutes after two. And the next thing I remember was I saw the clock again and it was five minutes to five and I was being sewn up. I remember being wheeled back to my room where my younger daughter and wife were waiting to greet me. They told me later I was very jovial and that they had looked at one another and said, 'He had surgery today and it was like nothing had happened to him.'

"The following day was quite different. I needed the morphine. But, you know, it wasn't the pain I was concerned about, it was the surgery. I was concerned about its success. But I heard nothing during the period I was in the hospital that gave me any reason to worry about it, and I would say, it wasn't that bad at all! I needed my report card! But I wouldn't get my report card back for several weeks to learn what my PSA was. But then I got word from Dr. Burnett, who told me the results were all very favorable. That was *good*!"

For Richard Meyers the results were better than good. He was and remains clear of prostate cancer and is free of incontinence and sexual dysfunction. Still, when he sees his fading abdominal scar in a mirror he is reminded of his brush with the disease and how he defeated it.

"The most difficult part of this process was the catheterization. I was very uncomfortable. It was the most terrible part of the experience, and it lasted only fourteen days. Even when I had the catheter removed, I didn't have any infection or anything like that, but still I was very uncomfortable and there was still some pain because the healing process had just not moved along enough, you know.

"So I started wearing some diapers and then I could switch over to wearing a pad inside my underwear. The urinary incontinence began to dissipate. I had urinary function in about ninety days. And I was dry! If I was sitting too long or I was in the car, I might get a leakage or a little squirt, but that was about it. Finally, all the leakage was gone and I was absolutely dry. I have no urinary problems whatsoever. My urinary function today is probably as good as it was when I was forty years old, as opposed to what it was before I had this surgery. My sexual function returned in maybe nine months. And when I started to see it happen without the Viagra [postsurgery], I started to feel like things were changing. And maybe it was as simple as when I would wake up in the morning and I had an erection or something that felt like an erection. But you know, it came back slowly and it continued to improve. So I would say that after about a year and a half I was feeling that I was at least ninety percent of the way there. Shortly thereafter, I was actually able to have intercourse *without Viagra!*"

Richard Meyers is keenly aware of his good fortune. He shares these thoughts with other men whose outcomes may not have been as providential as his. "If the cancer is out of your body you should consider yourself fortunate, whatever other issues you have to deal with, whether it's urinary or sexual dysfunction. As long as the cancer is gone, try to figure out how to get on with your life and make the best deal of it. Medical advances continue to be made. Look for other options. You just don't give up. I would continue to look for other alternatives of treatment and other ways to take care of yourself. You just never give up."

Richard Meyers, the survivor, is back on his bike, resuming his rigorous 180-mile treks between Philadelphia and the Jersey shore. He says his prostatectomy hasn't slowed him down a bit. He says biking gives him that full mind and body kind of workout that he really needs and enjoys.

The Doctor's Notebook

The testimonial of Richard Meyers would indicate the good fortune he had, but I would like to think his favorable outcome was not a matter of luck. My sense is that it was owed to his proper preparation. Upon being told of his diagnosis, he laboriously studied about his disease state, evaluated options, weighed advantages and disadvantages associated with these options, and then made an informed decision. In essence, he took charge of the matter and helped influence his own fate.

This level of responsibility in my patients is truly cherished. I appreciate their active decision making. This shows that they understand the actual goals, possibilities, and limitations of our current treatments. Also, they properly set expectations about what usually can be met. By his testimonial, I connect with his level of maturity in judgment. We fight this disease together, patient and surgeon. I have no more unrealistic sense of what we can accomplish than what my training and experience affords me. I am pleased to bring to patients my very best abilities and knowledge in providing them my best care. I attribute these circumstances to excellent outcomes for my patients, never thinking to pat myself on the back too hard when they do very well. Good fortune, for both him and me, is a consequence of preparedness and sensible action.

4

Malcolm "Mac" Ogilvie and Trudy Ogilvie

Don't Let Your Health Insurance Kill You!

Mac Ogilvie was a colonel in the U.S. Marine Corps and served his country for twenty-six years before retiring from the service. For the past twelve years he has been a math teacher and athletic coach at the James Fenimore Cooper Middle School in McLean, Virginia. He and his wife, Trudy, live in Springfield, Virginia, about an hour's drive from Washington, D.C. At the time of this interview he was fifty-nine. Mac is a pleasant, engaging, and slightly balding man with blue eyes. His children tease him, insisting he has but four hairs left on his head. Trudy is an ashy blonde with what her husband describes as "great legs."

Malcolm Ogilvie's health maintenance organization (HMO) failed to inform him that his PSA numbers were relatively high and were continuing to rise. In June 2005, his HMO physician performed a digital rectal exam (DRE) and felt a suspicious bulge on his prostate, then did a PSA, which turned out to be 6.8. His Gleason score was 7. The doctor then checked back over his records and told him his PSAs taken the previous three years were outside the safe range.

"When I heard that, I figured I was about two years late! I liked my doctor, but at the same time I realized he screwed up. I'd known people who found out they had cancer early and who had surgery, and they said if you get it early, it is treatable. So I was hoping I could have surgery. But then the surgeon at my health organization said, 'I don't think I'd recommend surgery. I think it's too late for you!' That's when I decided to visit a number of other urologists. One of them was in my same health organization. He told me he thought I need to be ready to look at chronic long-term cancer!

"If you go to the Partin tables [statistical data forecasting the stage of cancer spread], for people who had my 6.8 PSA and 7 Gleason score, there's a seventy-five percent chance the cancer has already spread beyond the prostate gland. So that means there's only a twenty-five percent chance of getting out of this without having chronic cancer.

"First thing I did was talk to friends to get ideas. I got hold of Dr. Patrick Walsh's book on prostate cancer [*Dr. Patrick Walsh's Guide to Surviving Prostate Cancer*] and read it cover to cover. And that was a very helpful book. I read other medical books. Everything that could get me up to speed. I went online and got sources on there for information really to figure out what was going on. I went to a support group over at Fairfax Hospital and heard different people in my same circumstances who *did* get rid of the cancer. And some that did *not* get rid of the cancer."

Then suddenly Mac got more bad news. He found out that he was also prediabetic. "Diabetes is not something to mess around with either. And I went on a very strict no-sugar diet—low-carb diet—and I worked out every day and I was much more careful about what I ate. Within six months I had lowered my sugar, but it's an ongoing thing I have to deal with—continually.

"So after all this, I went to see some other urologists. Some were willing to do the surgery, but they all thought I was at risk and told me they thought my chances of a favorable outcome were already gone. At that point, I went to Walter Reed, having been in the military. The doctors at Walter Reed compared whatever they were doing to Johns Hopkins. Hopkins does this,

Hopkins does that, and Hopkins gets results. It became obvious that they considered Johns Hopkins to be the gold standard when it came to prostate care. And that's when I made the decision to go to Hopkins.

"There, I met Dr. Arthur Burnett. He was the first to say I *was* a candidate for surgery. He does a ton of these operations. And he thought he could feel some clearance between the cancerous lumps of the prostate gland and the pelvic sidewall! So he judged that the cancerous lumps had not yet grown into the pelvic sidewall. If that was the case, Dr. Burnett explained, it would be an inoperative situation. I wanted a doctor who had a lot of experience. If a doctor doesn't hook you up right, he can totally foul you up. You can have real problems with incontinence or rectal problems. I know several people this has happened to. These life-and-death issues are tough. You're dealing with your own mortality, which is a difficult thing for everyone to deal with. I had been waking up every day with the thought that I had cancer in me and it might affect me in a long-term way and shorten my life. I sensed Dr. Burnett's confidence when he said he felt I had a chance. I needed to hear that. That's when I told him I'm ready to go for it." Surgery was set for November 22, 2005.

Mac Ogilvie conveyed his decision to his HMO. They told him they would not pay for the Hopkins surgery. Instead, they recommended that Mac let *them* do radiation. He rejected their advice and made arrangements to proceed with the surgery. "I looked at it and thought, hey, I'm in trouble here because of them. I thought I had a little legal case here. Meantime, I decided to pay for the whole thing myself. It turned out to be a huge bill, but I understood that from the get-go, so I didn't have any qualms about it. It's a lot of money, but I thought later I just might have a little talk with a lawyer.

"My wife, Trudy, throughout was very supportive. We've been through some difficult times in the past. Before I had my cancer, Trudy was afflicted with a virus that caused a condition called transverse myelitis. She became paralyzed below her waist, and so was confined to a wheelchair. She's now just beginning to walk again. But she's been through an incredible ordeal, and I've been supportive of everything she needed. And ever since I got this cancer, she's been totally supportive of me. We just felt our overall health issues were our paramount objectives. All the other things we were ready to work through. Before the surgery I said to Dr. Burnett, 'My intention is to have you do everything you can do to get rid of the cancer. That's number one. I would like to have the nerves spared, of course, but not if there is the slightest chance the cancer might spread. I mean I just wanted it gone.'"

The Ogilvies waited until March 15 to get the news they were waiting and hoping for. Mac's PSA registered 0.1, indicating that the cancer was no longer present. Dr. Burnett confirmed the success of the surgery. Surgical margins and lymph nodes: negative.

"It's now about four months since my operation. And I think the incontinence problem is pretty much over. I'm not sure I'm a hundred percent, but it's not a major issue. I do wear a small pad, but I'm not changing them several times a day anymore. As for the nerve bundles, Dr. Burnett felt if he did not take them, it could have resulted in retaining the cancer in me and he was with me on that—it was not even a chance he was willing to take. My family doctor says if you have a penis, you can have an erection. You're not going to be able to do it on your own, but it can be done. Pills, like Viagra, don't work for me, but I know there are other ways it can be done. Some are easier than others, and I'm going to look into those and we'll see. It's a factor, but not a huge factor. Not something totally distressing to me. I can deal with it. I'm utterly relieved that the cancer appears to be gone. Everything else is, I think, icing on the cake. And my wife's and my relationship is not based one hundred percent on our sexual ability in that manner. There are so many other ways we share a closeness and emotions together."

Mac Ogilvie is a man who is quite philosophical about life. When he talks about his recent ordeal, he likes to reflect on the lessons it has taught him. "You know, as men get older, they lose a certain level of their sexual potency and capability. And when you see what can potentially happen with radiation treatment for prostate cancer or radical surgery—with or without the loss of the nerve bundles—eventually you still lose potency. You know, my knees have aged and I can't use my knees as well as I used to.

Same thing with sexual function. I think I could reconcile that in my own mind. Other people may or may not.

"I discovered that when I went to some of the support groups, they were very helpful. You meet other people in the same exact situation and you become very close to them because you're all really facing the same things. And your faith could also be a strength for you. It could be a source of comfort and reconciliation of your situation. I think the human mind and body is able to try coping with things. After you go through the period where you just feel bad for yourself—and all the different levels of grief for yourself—I think, in the long run, you are able to adjust and cope with your new situation. And I think that's what life is all about, in a way. Adjusting to new situations. For whatever reason, I think I am very fortunate—lucky. I was one of those twenty-five percent who made it. I'll be ever thankful and try to make the rest of my life worthwhile for having deserved to be free of cancer. I tell people, 'If you ever see me not smiling, you have my permission to hit me on the side of the head, because I ought to be smiling all the time.'"

Perhaps nothing sustains Mac Ogilvie in all he does and accomplishes more than the love and encouragement of his wife, Trudy. She is, he will tell you, his rock and the source of his inspiration. Trudy Ogilvie works with fifth-graders as a special-needs computer teacher. When he came home one day and told her he might have prostate cancer, she was jolted: "He said he had to wait for a biopsy report to come back, but he added there was little doubt that he had it. Mac takes very good care of himself. He had a physical every year. We both tried over the past couple of years to eat better, change our habits. Exercise is very crucial now, so it was a *shock* that this was not caught by his HMO doctors! His PSA would go to that level and nobody noticed it! Mac's physician at their HMO, Dr. Gallagher, was the nicest of doctors. But Mac was so angry at him. He had had so much respect for him and yet he screwed up—and because of that Mac was facing cancer. Both of his parents died of cancer. So this was a very real threat. It was devastating. It was because of *you*, Dr. Gallagher—you screwed up—my whole life is changed forever!

"We have four children. The oldest is thirty-three and the youngest twenty-three, and we're all very close. At first, I didn't want to tell them about Mac because they were scattered all over the country and I knew it was going to be devastating for them. But we always made a promise after what had happened to me, when I got transverse myelitis, that we would never, never keep anything from one another—never, never! That was our promise. Our family had been through so much with me, and very, very supportive. So, now this. My heart just broke for Mac. I just started praying. I'm a Catholic and raised Irish Catholic. And my faith has got me through many, many things. That's where I go! That's my end. I just prayed. Every day. I believe we're here for a reason and it's for each other. And Mac got me through it all with his sense of humor. With his joking around. He can take a really delicate situation and make me laugh.

"Communication is crucial at a time like this. You have to have someone to talk to. You have to sort of vent. I have very close friends, but it was sort of between Mac and me. I mean, we spoke about what was going to be happening and all, but I didn't really get into the gravity of it all. I had to deal with it with my kids first. You know, they were devastated and I felt like a walking sob story. So we kept it between us. Our relationship just got stronger. All of a sudden we realized what was important in our lives. We just want to enjoy life. We want to enjoy our kids. We want to enjoy people. *Things* don't mean anything. Your faith in God and a belief that you're loved, I think, is the most important thing that life has to offer you. It makes you open up more to other people much easier. You're not afraid. Here I am! This is *me*! When you're in your thirties and forties, you want to be liked. You want this, you want that. When you're in your fifties and sixties, you just want your mate by your side for the rest of your life! We do have so much fun together."

Malcolm Ogilvie made good on his promise to visit his lawyer. He drafted a letter of complaint to his HMO and within two weeks received notice that they had reversed their decision. He says the letter that ended with "Your referral is approved" made his day. When last contacted, he was in the process of collecting $19,000 from his HMO.

The Doctor's Notebook

This is an extremely touching story. Malcolm Ogilvie and his wife, Trudy, had presented to me in a state of hopelessness and despair because of his prostate cancer diagnosis. Additionally, I could sense their anger as they were told they had a situation that had progressed despite his good health maintenance activities. Nevertheless, we were determined in moving forward with the radical prostatectomy, and ultimately he had a success story. His epiphany is that he should be "smiling all the time" because of his positive outcome. This perception actually shows Mac's upbeat spirit despite having gone through his ordeal. His account reveals how much anxiety and emotional upheaval this disease can produce.

In my encounter with the Ogilvies, my own sense of anxiety also was elevated. I too was disappointed that Mac's clinical condition had progressed in such a way that his very best outcome, disease eradication with preservation of functional abilities to the fullest extent, might be compromised. Our interconnection was direct and honest, as we both understood the gravity of his situation. Also, I had some deep concerns about how likely we were to beat the odds. The extent of his local disease was unclear and therefore very disconcerting. How much intrusion had the cancer made beyond the prostate capsule? This admission of angst from my perspective reflects how much we physicians may agonize over achieving the very best results for our patients. In the final analysis, I reasoned that the odds in Mac Ogilvie's situation were somewhat unfavorable. Yet as I examined his case, I came to the conclusion that because of my training and experience, he had a chance. And so we proceeded. The outcome, happily, was quite positive, and I am smiling with him.

There are some additional insights gained from Mac Ogilvie's story. Indeed, his case demonstrates a late diagnosis. This situation can occur, but it is avoidable. It is known that prostate cancer kills, and great responsibility should be borne by all involved, including patients themselves, in coming to grips with this fact and in taking a leading role in their own care. It is a tribute to both Mac and Trudy Ogilvie that they were persistent in his management. He was not prepared to accept anything less than a reasonable attempt to be successful. An additional observation associated with this energy is his wife's extremely supportive stance. A physician should never forget that we learn much from our patients about life's lessons. Experiences such as this are gratifying for me, while they also reaffirm my purpose in becoming a physician.

Prescriptive Information

About Surgery

We speak of surgery as the "gold standard" because it is the premier method of curing patients of prostate cancer. Using the PSA test, we are able to find prostate cancers while they are small and contained within the prostate capsule. If cancer is discovered in a healthy man who has a potentially long life ahead of him, surgery offers an excellent way of ridding the patient of the cancer for good!

The prevailing prostate surgical procedure carried out in our major cancer centers is the radical prostatectomy. It involves the complete removal of the prostate gland and surrounding tissue, including the seminal vesicles. Why not remove only the prostate gland? The answer is that prostate cancer pops up in several areas inside the prostate at once. Surgeons refer to that as "multifocal." We still don't have instruments that are accurate enough to pinpoint where those little tumors are, and for the most part they are too tiny to be discovered during a DRE. Even if we could remove the central focus of the cancer in the prostate, the very small cancerous tumors could eventually grow, metastasize, and disperse elsewhere where detection would be almost impossible. So surgeons opt to remove the entire gland, together with surrounding tissue, in an attempt to forestall future spread of the cancer. While carrying out the procedure, skilled surgeons work to minimize heavy bleeding and prevent urinary complications. At the same time, they will make the all-important judgment call about whether they can perform nerve-sparing surgery (preventing damage to the erectile nerves), thereby preserving sexual function. It is a call based primarily on curing the patient's cancer and avoiding a future recurrence of the disease.

Many experts describe the ideal candidate for a radical prostatectomy as a man in his forties or early fifties, in good health, and with good sexual and urinary function. That said, there are those, like Dr. Arthur Burnett, who believe you can't pigeonhole men who don't fall strictly within those boundaries. They strongly hold to the opinion that age alone need not be a barrier to surgery. If an older man is in excellent health and in excellent physical condition with expectations of considerable longevity—perhaps ten to twenty years—he should not be ruled out as a candidate. Rather, the determination should be made, say Dr. Burnett and his colleagues, on the basis of careful clinical examination and psychologically pertinent factors, not defined strictly by chronological age. In short, men beyond the age of fifty in good physical condition with perceived longevity may well pass the qualifications for a successful radical prostatectomy.

The Radical Prostatectomy

Commonly asked questions about surgery include the following:

"Will surgery cure my cancer?"

"If I choose surgery, will I lose my ability to have sex?"

"How do I go about choosing the right surgeon?"

"What are my risks choosing surgery?"

Early surgical procedures used a procedure called a perineal prostatectomy. An incision was made behind the scrotal sac. The problem was that the surgeon's view of the crucial structures within was extremely limited by the narrow "porthole window" he worked in. The results were greatly disappointing. Even though patients made quick recoveries, they were left with incontinence and sexual dysfunction. Today, experienced surgeons have moved light-years ahead, performing what they call a radical prostatectomy. The technique involves making a vertical abdominal incision that provides a clear view of the operating field. It allows the surgeon easy access to the prostate as well as all nearby vital organs and tissues. The procedure gives patients a fighting chance to do away with cancer for good, preserve their potency, eliminate incontinence, and resume their normal lives. If a patient decides to undergo surgery, he should be certain to ask his doctor whether the doctor can perform the more acceptable nerve-sparing radical prostatectomy, a far better choice when it comes to preserving sexual function and providing the best all-around outcome.

Many doctors today are using an innovative surgical procedure called laparoscopic surgery. They remove the prostate using high-tech microsurgical instrumentation. Laparoscopy uses a lighted tube that enters the body through a tiny hole and through which the surgeon can thread a scalpel. The surgical field is magnified and projected onto a monitor, providing an excellent view of internal structures. The abdomen is then inflated with gas to make room for insertion of the surgical instruments. Those who perform these operations say the procedure offers the advantages of less bleeding and the ability to make a watertight connection. More recently a robot connected to special instruments has taken laparoscopic surgery to the next level, providing new surgical refinements.

The reader should know that according to the *Cancer Journal for Clinicians* (September 2009), laparoscopic surgical techniques have not been proven to produce better erection recovery than open radical prostatectomy. No long-term studies are yet available to determine if laparoscopic procedures offer the same rate of cancer control as a radical prostatectomy. Nonetheless, competent, experienced surgeons presumably all have one goal in common: to do the surgery as best they can with proper, complete prostate removal while minimizing trauma to the nerves that control sexual function.

Those who practice laparoscopic/robotic surgery say the scars are tiny compared to the three- to four-inch incisions in the open prostatectomy, and hospital stays are shorter. Skilled surgeons are required to perform the procedure. Inexperience can lead to serious complications, requiring conversion to an open procedure midstream to stop blood loss or damage to an injured organ. One stated major downside to laparoscopic/robotic surgery at the moment is that it doesn't allow the surgeon the tactile sensation he or she would like during the nerve-sparing procedure; the surgeon is denied the ability to feel the tissue to make certain it is safe to preserve the nerves. Also, in the laparoscopic/robotic procedure, the doctor is unable to use his fingers to check for stickiness—a strong indicator that some cancer may still be present. In the final analysis, the successful outcome of prostate cancer surgery depends foremost on the ability of the doctor performing the surgery. This is true whether the procedure involves the open radical method or the laparoscopic and/or robotic-assisted laparoscopic techniques.

5

Paul Haley

For Some, Faith Can Illuminate the Obscure Decision-Making Process

Paul Haley is the director of planned giving at the U.S. Navy Memorial Foundation in Washington, D.C. The organization, mandated by Congress, is a nonprofit group dedicated to promoting naval history. Paul Haley is in charge of coordinating charitable gifts from individual donors.

There is an especially immaculate look about Paul's whole appearance, from his starched pale green shirt that matches the color of his eyes to his neatly combed light brown hair that's just beginning to gray. The rimless glasses he wears are nearly square, and he has a pleasant smile and an easy manner.

He lives alone in a small apartment in Alexandria, Virginia, overlooking richly endowed green lawns. The apartment itself is modest and spotless. Glance about, and the space is replete with artifacts of his faith. Paul Haley was sixty-four when we spoke with him, and when in 2003 he discovered he had prostate cancer, his reaction was not different from that of so many men.

"First I was shocked. I said to myself, 'Why *me*?' Then I was angry. You know why? Because I felt I should have been invited by my doctor to bring somebody with me. It was just me and the doctor. I felt he was in some way leading me to a decision.

The first thing I wanted to do was to get out of there! I needed to process what I had just been told. I didn't want to just sit there and listen to too much information in terms of what 'we' were going to do next.

"I had nobody in my family with prostate cancer, so my reaction was one of total surprise. I can't say at that moment I was scared. That came later. But I'll tell you the scary part. It was that I had never been in a hospital in my whole life! I had never gone under anesthesia. In fact, I had never spent a single overnight in a hospital. I just could not fathom the fact that somewhere down the road this was going to involve surgery, and this was going to involve time in a hospital. And *my God*! That was just too much for me to even deal with.

"I had no symptoms at all. But the doctor told me that over two and a half years my PSA level had about doubled, starting in the 2s and getting into the early 4s. And I was pretty aware that when the PSA jumps like that it's a significant change. And so this doctor suggested it was time to get a biopsy. I had no symptoms, but I had the biopsy because my physician suggested it get done. Two weeks later the results came back, and I found myself in my urologist's office being told, yes, I did have prostate cancer. As I say, I was angry and it came as a complete surprise. Now, I am a very prayerful person. And I find that when I take whatever the situation is and step away from it and reflect on it, I personally find it easier to deal with."

Like many others in his position, Paul decided to pull some information together. The doctor had given him a book on prostate cancer. Paul did some research online and talked to people he knew, in particular a very close friend, who would go with him to the urologist's for the follow-up visit two weeks later. "When we got there, the entire tone of the conversation changed. The doctor's persona changed. And I decided that my mission was to encourage general practitioners *never* to send a man in to receive news—whether good news or bad news—by himself! I had brought another person with me who was not just listening to the doctor, but another person who would be a listening partner for me as I approached a decision. And so what got on the table were questions I wasn't even prepared to ask during the first visit.

Such as: How often do you do this surgery? What do you think about the hospital that you are connected with? What are some of the alternatives and what do you think of those alternatives? When the doctor told us on average he usually did one operation a month, maybe two, I wasn't getting to a comfort level. The only thing going through my head was I wouldn't buy a cake from a cake decorator that only decorated one cake a month, why should I turn my body over to somebody who is performing major surgery only once or twice a month? And when he admitted he didn't do nerve sparing because he hadn't taken the time to learn, I knew this doctor was not on top of his game, and told my general practitioner the same.

"I was exploring radiation, but all of a sudden I felt as though I had my back against the wall. So at this point I decided to talk to folks outside the area. I spoke with two friends in Boston who had the disease. One had seed implants. He chose that in combination with radiation because he has a heart condition, and it has worked fantastically for him. One did surgery, and that's worked out well for him. In gathering information about radiation, I realized that there were new techniques that were very much refined. Pinpoint laser devices where radiation is delivered exactly where it's supposed to be delivered, as opposed to the old practice of delivering it to a general area. And it's controlled in an appropriate manner that's very effective with some individuals.

"I decided to look further at seed implants, but in my case, that was not going to happen because my prostate was enlarged. Another step had to take place first. Basically, it would mean I would have to have hormone shots or pills, whatever, to reduce the size of the prostate. And so at this point I realized the decision was going to have to be mine and mine alone.

"I have a personal relationship with the Lord that enables me to come to a decision in the unbelievable speed of light. And I knew that I wasn't going to overcome my dilemma until I had at least taken some baby steps to get to the point that when that insight came, I would have a little background as to the larger comment.

"Within a few weeks from the second visit to the urologist, I went on a business trip to Chicago. And during some downtime,

I met a very close friend who was a cancer survivor. That morning he took me to visit the cathedral in Chicago, and that's when I basically presented my case to the Lord, as to what I had gathered [in the way of information] and where we should be going from there. As I was just getting ready to leave the cathedral, I said, 'Lord, I am not hearing anything.' And there it was in my mind! The word 'cut'! As simple as that, I walked out of there, knowing that no matter how much dancing around the issue I might do, no matter how much I was to pursue the possibility of seed implants, there was no way of getting around it. The Lord had spoken and that was the action to take. Immediately I started asking questions about the top places in the country with regard to prostate surgery. I got input from a brother in Boston who provides accounting services to most of the hospitals in the city. He picked up the phone, called a client, and asked him, 'If you had to make one hospital choice in the United States, what would it be?' The answer was Hopkins. That was all I needed to hear.

"My appointment was set for the end of January in 2004. In the time leading up to that date, I was so impressed with all the steps that had to take place for my appointment with my surgeon, Dr. Burnett. I had to present tissue slides from my urologist. I needed to go online and fill out forms. It was all so very well facilitated. I had not run into any medical situations before where it was so smooth and coordinated.

"The hardest thing was to accept the fact that I was going to be put under and I was going to be operated on. Those were my two anxieties because I'm a person who's always in control. Who knows what you might do while you're coming out of anesthesia? I envisioned waking up and pulling plugs out of myself, and I needed somebody to tell me there was going to be somebody there to help.

"But the reality was that everything went well. Looking back, I would have liked it if somebody had talked me through all that in advance. It might have been helpful, just to know what the experience was going to be. There was a great sense of relief when I did wake up there. And a nurse told me everything had gone well. Within twenty minutes the doctor himself came by to tell me, 'I feel everything went well with the surgery. We'll have some test results back in a few days.'

"I guess I really didn't anticipate that whole business with the catheter. I would have liked to have been prepped to know I would be walking around with that for fourteen days or so and that I had to stay in the hospital until my bowels came back to function. Within two and a half days that was back in action! There was a lot of housekeeping stuff nobody had talked about until now. Like how to change the urine bag for the catheter. After the catheter came out I learned that I was going to have to wear sanitary pads in my underwear. I was going to be doing a lot of experimenting with my urinary incontinence. I had to be very proactive. My quick decision was, well, forget all the hunt-and-peck nonsense with pads; just wear the disposable underwear! It made it so much better, and it took me two weeks to figure that out. Disposable underwear was the way to go, and there would be no mishaps, mistakes, whatever. But after a certain period of time, I wasn't urinating at random. After four months I was able to switch from disposable underwear to medium pads. Today, I still use a very small disposable pad. But that's my personal preference so I won't be surprised in case there is some small amount of leakage that could occur randomly, infrequently."

As for sexual function, Paul is now able to get a full erection. One of the reasons that he chose Johns Hopkins was that his surgeon used the nerve-sparing technique. "I felt if I was going to go for the surgery, I was going to go for the best. It was not an issue because of marriage or sexual function. It was simply if what is being delivered is the best, then that's what I'm going to go for. I am single. I am not sexually active. That was not a part, but I figured if they're offering something that might be important to me at another point in time, then I'm going to go for that.

"I've been very honest about everything I've had to deal with. And I found my surgeon available. *Always* available. My strategy for coping is to be brutally honest. If I felt I might have some leakage, for whatever reason—too much coffee, too much alcohol, whatever—then I know what I need to do in terms of underwear pads. So there are no surprises. I always carry a couple of extra pads with me in my briefcase. I'm aware that if I swim, I need to urinate before I leave the pool area—because that exercise seems to precipitate a little leakage, I can easily fix that problem. There's always a little pad for protection.

"I've found that each time I've gone to see Dr. Burnett at Hopkins, I've ended up sharing with one of his patients. They may be in a different situation than I'm in. Most of them have either had surgery or are about to have it. It's made me realize how important it is to share concerns and experiences, to get some feelings out on the table that maybe are still ruminating in your mind. Communication is vital." Paul Haley is a man who is happy with his work. He vows never to retire because, he says, he is just having too much fun.

The Doctor's Notebook

Paul Haley tells an uplifting story that is consistent with his effervescent personality. His story in many respects parallels others in that he experienced a mix of emotions: surprise, anger, fear, anxiety, and frank honesty. His manner of dealing with his prostate cancer diagnosis was to open lines of communication. He remarks on the importance of a "listening partner" when consulting with the physician, to get all of the information correctly and discuss all possible issues. I believe in this approach as well. It is a routine of my practice that I always call my patients for a brief telephone chat about a week after they have seen me initially. I inform them after they leave me the first time that I want them to have the opportunity to consider all issues that may not come to them initially, discuss all matters with chosen individuals at home, and be ready to ask me any question whatsoever to allay their fears and anxieties.

Paul Haley also speaks to various other strategies that worked for him in arriving at his best decision for treatment. He is a very religious person, and prayer and faith absolutely mattered. He took personal responsibility for his decision to try to avoid potential problems, and to be sure that he was getting the very best care.

This insight is enlightening, but at the same time it is not a new concept. In fact, not all health-care providers—or surgeons, for that matter—are the same in terms of training, experience, ability, availability, and most important, interest in the patient. All of these characteristics matter to me. I believe it should matter to patients. Paul Haley's comments should remind all patients to find a good communicative surgeon and one who meets *all* of the qualifications that matter to them.

6

Russell Windle and Victor Kralisz

Gay Men and Prostate Cancer: Invisible Burdens

To hear Russell Windle tell it, as recently as 2001, he was the first gay person to post on the prostate support Web site You Are Not Alone Now (www.yananow.net). He checked other sites and concluded that prostate support groups for the gay community were practically nonexistent. So Russell Windle started his own. He called it Prostate Cancer and Gay Men, a site he set up on Yahoo (http://health.groups.yahoo.com/group/prostatecancerandgaymen/). Since then, others have come along, a number of which have affiliated with his.

Russell was simply following his own philosophy of helping others. In 2001, he became a prostate cancer survivor. That "miracle" was sufficient to ignite his personal sense of obligation to offer help and support to other men diagnosed with the disease, particularly gay men who felt cut off from society and alone, with no sense of where to turn.

Russell Windle is a technical writer in the medical division of Olympus America, Inc. He writes user guides for chemical and blood bank analyzers—much of the equipment, he explains, required in the testing of PSAs. Russell is an engaging, highly intelligent man, heavyset, tall, with dark brown hair, a full beard, and blue eyes. He wears glasses and laughs easily. Russell lives in Dallas with his partner, Victor Kralisz. When we spoke with Russell in May 2008, he was fifty-seven.

Victor Kralisz is the manager of the arts and humanities department at the main public library in downtown Dallas. Victor has a professorial look about him. He is lean with a salt-and-pepper beard, wears thin silver-framed glasses, and speaks softly with a sonorous baritone voice. At the time of this interview, Victor was sixty-two.

Russell admittedly is not much of a sports fan, but he will tell you that he always loved to go swimming and bowling. He also liked taking long walks and being active, and he has tried to stay in good physical shape. When he turned forty, he thought it was time to begin having regular physicals. "I tried to have them every year, but sometimes I'd miss. It got to be every two or three years. When I turned fifty, I thought I should be more diligent. So I went in for my physical. Dr. Brooks took my vitals, drew some blood to measure my PSA, and said he wanted to do a DRE. When he did that, he told me he felt a lump on the prostate wall. We waited for the lab results to come back, and that's when Dr. Brooks told me that my PSA was 5.2. He said it could be an indication of prostate cancer, and he wanted me to see a urologist. He made the appointment, and I went to see the urologist, Dr. Ross."

Russell chose Dr. Brooks as his internist first because he knew him to be an excellent physician, and second because he knew Dr. Brooks was gay. Why did Russell consider the doctor's sexual orientation so important? "My preference was because I wanted a doctor I could be completely open with. I wanted no facet of my life to be hidden from him. If I came down with hepatitis, he'd know why. And in this area, especially Dallas, it's ultra-conservative and ultra–religious right. By choosing a gay physician, I don't have to deal with all the narrow-mindedness. When it came to my having to see a urologist, I told Dr. Brooks I preferred a gay urologist. And he said, 'The doctor I'm sending you to, Dr. Ross, is not gay. But he is gay-friendly.' And that promised to work for me."

"Dr. Ross did the DRE again, and he felt the same lump on the right lobe of the prostate. He also said my prostate was enlarged and my bladder was overextended. He put me on Flomax and told me to come back in a week."

The urologist's finding of the enlarged prostate would help explain the symptoms Russell had been experiencing for some time prior to his physical exam by Dr. Brooks. "I was having frequent urination. I'd get up five, six, maybe seven times during the night. And I couldn't drive from home to work without stopping to go to the bathroom. If I went on long trips, it would add about an hour to the trip because I'd have to go to the bathroom. I mean, it was really urgent and frequent."

The following week when Russell returned for a follow-up, the urologist repeated the digital rectal exam, and performed a sonogram of the bladder. "Then he told me he wanted to do a biopsy, and so he made the arrangement for the following Friday. On January 31, 2001, at nine-fifty in the morning—that's when I got the news. I had a malignant tumor on the right side of my prostate!

"Right then I wasn't upset about it. I called my uncle Bill. He said, 'You're a Windle, you have blue eyes, you're a male—you're gonna have prostate problems. We males in the family all have prostate problems.' The men in my family have BPH and high PSA readings. But it turned out I was the first Windle to have prostate cancer! I was horrified. I was terrified. Dr. Ross tried to reassure me. He said there's a fifty-fifty chance that the cancer is still encapsulated. I went home and cried and screamed and hurt. But then I managed to pull myself together and decided I needed to go out and take my mind off of the cancer. Since I was about to move, I loaded up my pickup and began moving my things into my new apartment."

A few days later, Russell sat down with his urologist to hear about his options. "Dr. Ross expressed the hope that the cancer had been caught in time. He was very open about it all as he talked about the options and potential risks. I could either have surgery or radiation. When he talked about radiation he told me there was a risk of recurrence. He also pointed out that with surgery there's always a chance one little cell could escape and cause a recurrence down the line. I just wanted the damned thing out of my body, and I didn't want to revisit this down the line."

Russell did research. He says he searched the Internet to find out as much as he could about the options, and he pored over some medical texts. In the end, he chose to have a radical prostatectomy. "I had my procedure done at Medical City, a private hospital here in Dallas. But I have to tell you, I was terrified about going in for the operation. Dr. Ross was recommended very highly and he had done tons of operations. I remember being scared to death before they put me under. And just before, I muttered to myself, 'I can fly . . . I can die . . . so let's get this thing over with.' The surgery itself took about three hours. The very next morning when I sat up I could feel the staples in my abdomen. Boy, did that hurt! I didn't have time to focus much on that because the next thing I knew they attached my IV to a pole and had me up and walking. I was a little rocky at first and sat down to regain my strength. But when I got up again, I managed to walk around the whole corridor that made a square around the hospital. The next day I got released—it was a Saturday—and I felt a little uncomfortable because I was dragging a catheter along with me.

"Initially, I had what Dr. Ross called stress incontinence. When they took the catheter out, I expected to flood, but I never had any serious incontinence! Dr. Ross told me how amazing that was. I just had a little dribble. I was dry three weeks after the operation! In fact, at night I didn't have to sleep with a pad at all."

Dr. Ross was able to save both of Russell's nerve bundles. "When doctors reviewed the pathology report, they found the cancer was indeed confined to the prostate itself. It had gone from the right side over to the left side, but had never escaped the capsule. Dr. Ross said there was a fifty-fifty chance that they'd caught it in time." It's seven years now since the surgery, and Russell is clear of cancer. "The erection is okay, but it's not constant. I had no luck with natural erections until eighteen months after my surgery. Three months after surgery, I was using a VED [vacuum erection device]. It was good . . . I mean better than nothing. I could pump it up, so to speak. And I remember the first orgasm I had the first time I pumped it up. But it hurt and I was told that it was because of fibrosis, those are the little fibers that grow into the caverns controlling erections. They engorge with blood when you're getting an erection. Later I found that if I use Levitra or one of the other ED [erectile dysfunction] drugs, [my ability to get an erection is] excellent, but getting it on my own? I can get it there, but not to the extent I can with Levitra. So I think the nerves are still regenerating. So, I take it one day at a time. I don't want to rush it."

However, there is more than just the physical aspect. How did Russell handle the emotional and psychological consequences? "At first I felt distraught. I began feeling like less than a person. I felt like used goods. Nobody would want me for that aspect. And then I got to thinking, 'If that's all they want with me, then do I really want them?' That's when Victor came into my life, and he became a permanent fixture. I was using the pump at the time, and we would use the pump as foreplay."

What lessons can Russell Windle pass on to gay men or heterosexual men from his experience in battling prostate cancer? "I tell them the three Rs: relax, research, and react. Research what you're gonna have done. I did it. Once I got out of Dr. Ross's office, I went straight onto the Internet and looked up all kinds of therapies. And I also looked up the consequences of recurrence. I got some books, including the Walsh book [*Dr. Patrick Walsh's Guide to Surviving Prostate Cancer*].

"For instance, I learned that with radiation, while I might not be incontinent or impotent to begin with, three to five years later cancer can recur. When I consulted with an oncologist, he never told me I could be impotent after radiation or there could be internal bleeding. So be your own advocate. Research! Research! React! That's my advice."

After his operation, Russell found it was his calling to reach out to others who also needed help. He said it was just ridiculous that the need for a gay support group was not being met by somebody, so he started his blog, Prostate Cancer and Gay Men.

"I talked to a lot of guys on my site and I hear a lot of horror stories: 'I am six months out [from my operation] and I'm still flooding.' 'I have no control.' I can only thank my lucky stars that I escaped those problems. [Before I set up my site] I found support groups were very important. I got onto You Are Not Alone Now, where I made my post. I was the first gay man there to mention my sexual orientation. I did some posts on Phoenix 5 too, but in

March 2001, the same year that I had my prostatectomy, I went online with my own blog.

"It's an interesting group. It started out with a number of straight men emailing me wanting to join the group. And I said, 'As long you respect us, we will respect you.' I have no problem with it. The men all talk freely about sexual matters, more than they could in other sites. We take off the gloves, so to speak.

"Many of these men either had a prostatectomy, are considering having one, or may be dealing with the effects of it. Or they're wanting to know about other therapies for prostate cancer. And there are also a number of women on my blog, and maybe two to three percent of the bloggers are women whose husbands have had or now have prostate cancer. Before I started my blog, I felt bad that there was no real outlet for gay men who were dealing with prostate cancer. It was just another closet that they were hiding in.

"A short time after I started my blog, Darryl Mitteldorf, a social worker who works for New York State, started a group he called Male Care, and he contacted me about associating his group with mine. And so I am on Male Care, too; our groups are affiliated with each other. Mitteldorf started other prostate cancer groups outside of major U.S. cities with an eye toward reaching gay men in rural areas, giving them a chance to talk with other gay men who are dealing with prostate cancer. Communication is a lot worse in rural areas than it is in big cities because you have to be secretive in small towns, whereas you can be as open as hell in big cities where nobody cares. My group alone now has members in Britain, New Zealand, Australia, and all around the world."

When it comes to the treatment of gay men with prostate cancer, are there special considerations their heterosexual physicians need to keep in mind? What are the obligations and expectations of the gay patient with respect to his heterosexual doctor? If a gay patient puts his life in the hands of a gay physician, does the relationship between the two really guarantee better outcomes?

"I think sometimes a problem exists that has as much to do with the gay patient as it has to do with his heterosexual physician. This happens when the gay man keeps secrets from his doctor.

Like, if I went to a doctor and told him I had an anal tear from having sex with my lover and he took umbrage to that, it would be the last time I would walk through his door. I'd find another physician who wouldn't be offended. But, you see, it's also the fault of the gay men who keep secrets from their doctors. Physicians may be open and have no problems with their gay patients. But then the problem starts when the gay man hides in the closet.

"And there's a particular problem that comes up with respect to gay doctors. These gay urologists often seem so desperate for their patients to have erections that they start talking to them about having implants about a year or less after they've had surgery. I know one who encourages patients to have artificial sphincters to cure incontinence and penile implants inserted for sexual activity six months after prostate surgery. Not waiting long enough to see if the incontinence will disappear naturally. Not waiting long enough to see if the erections will come back. A year can often be too soon. If incontinence is a real problem causing flooding constantly, I say, fine, you may have to look into that. But wait at least a year for the natural erection to come back. Assuming, of course, the patient still has his nerve bundles intact. I tell men that in some cases potency can take two or even three years to return. But once that implant is in, it can't be undone.

"When it comes to the question of whether there is a loss of sensitivity in anal penetration following a radical prostatectomy, I would have to respond this way. I do believe the answer is yes. I've found that there is a greater degree of sensitivity when the prostate is there. And I believe that if you remove it, there is less sensitivity. But it is nothing you can't live without. There are a lot of masseuses now that will give a prostate massage. And that's in the gay and straight worlds. So I suppose the sensitivity is there in both sexual orientations. Some of it may be lost when the prostate is removed. I'd also like to say that there were straight men in our blog group who allow penetration by their wives with a dildo. And they said they've found it very pleasurable. When they told me this, I said, 'Okay, you're telling me something we didn't know.' It was a shock to me that they realized it could be pleasurable. That's why I say that the straight and gay communities are just as sexually diverse. From my perspective, as long as it's not hurting anybody, well, that's fine."

Russell's partner, Victor, points to misunderstandings in society that color relationships between heterosexuals and gays alike, including physicians. "Many heterosexuals believe that when it comes to gays, their sole or primary concern centers on sex. Well, sex may be uppermost in the minds of some gay men, particularly young men. But there are multiple reasons why gay couples choose to live together. Bringing up children, for instance. Becoming active in their communities would be another. A lot of gay people are simply interested in establishing good relationships. This is one essential thing about gay people that so many people in our society, for whatever reason, simply don't understand."

Assuming a gay patient has had good outcomes following a radical prostatectomy—the cancer has been removed, continence has returned, nerves have been spared, and potency has returned—does the gay man have other issues, including possible psychological ones that are not shared by a heterosexual patient?

Russell says, "The only thing I can think of is that in the relationship with the primary care provider, problems can crop up if the gay patient doesn't let his sexual orientation be known to the doctor. They'll tell the doctor everything about themselves, but they won't come out. They won't say, 'I'm gay . . . I have this or that problem.' In my own case, I had a bit of depression after the surgery, but from what I've seen and understand, that is quite normal. You will have questions that come up from anywhere between six months to a year. I'm methodical in what I do. I never put myself in a position I don't want to be in. I wanted a gay primary care provider so I could talk to him openly about my sexual orientation and what I'm doing. I know there are a lot of men who put themselves through the wringer and they really don't have to, gay as well as straight."

What about the men who remain so anxious about their dwindling potency? What can Russell tell them?

"So many of them are in the position where they are either injecting or taking drugs or using pumps or a combination of those to get a 'good' erection. They should in my view relax and not put so much pressure on themselves to get hard."

Prostate cancer is a particularly stressful disease. Beyond the physical problems the patient has to face are the psychological ones that can be extremely profound. For all men there are the assaults on their virility and the effects on their lives and loved ones. Prostate cancer puts additional stress on our growing older population already burdened by society's obsession with eternal youth. It imposes stressful challenges on African American men who are far less able to undergo routine screening because of limited access to health care. But the psychological stress on gay men throughout the population is little understood in our predominately heterosexual population. We feel we would have been remiss in not acknowledging the special needs and concerns of gay men who have faced or will face the ravages of prostate cancer.

The Doctor's Notebook

The testimonials of Russell and his partner, Victor, are enlightening. Perhaps first and foremost is the revelation that the challenges and anxieties of a prostate cancer diagnosis and then proceeding with treatment affect all men similarly irrespective of sexual orientation. No doubt these gentlemen are wonderful human beings to tell their stories and to take such a proactive role in the war against prostate cancer. They attest their homosexual orientation while also stating that their experience supports the cause of men beyond this factor. At the same time, they both recognize the very important need to help gay men grapple with the personal effects of prostate cancer. I commend them to the highest level and value their contribution to this book.

Their overall message connects well with me as a physician. I strongly believe that we physicians should be faithful and respectful to patients. They divulge their most sensitive and personal matters to us, expecting trust and commitment and that any knowledge of intimate matters may help us provide them the very best care. In my opinion, physicians should interact without bias and with the highest intent of service no matter the circumstance, whether it be differing cultural background, religious beliefs, political ideology, or even sexual orientation. I will take the opportunity of this forum to further emphasize a point made by Russell and Victor. They acknowledge that we are all human beings with common human frailties. Indeed, although there may be diverse personalities, interests, and styles characterizing all of us, we are more alike than different. Our likeness relates to our humanness, and in the matter of prostate cancer the disease makes no distinctions about its potential to claim lives. Their message, which I support, is to overcome ignorance and be supportive of each other.

I appreciate the concerns of sexual function recovery in gay men undergoing treatment for prostate cancer. The matter of sexual function recovery following radical prostatectomy is hardly minor for men undergoing this surgery, and perhaps special appreciation is owed to those who are able to be fully open and forthright about discussing and addressing it. The effect of prostate cancer treatments, including radical prostatectomy, on sexual function for the patient and partner cannot be overemphasized. The impact may relate not only to erectile function but also ejaculatory function and libido. It may be true that we urologists have not given enough attention to all the matters of sexual function that could be compromised following treatment for prostate cancer.

Both Russell and Victor correctly acknowledge the importance of "nerve sparing" that may be performed at the time of radical prostatectomy. This term refers to the nerves coursing around the prostate that terminate in the penis and govern the erectile response necessary for erection. The goal of the urologic surgeon is to maximize functional recovery in all respects with radical prostatectomy. However, nerve preservation should not come at the cost of incomplete cancer removal in an unfortunate patient whose cancer may be locally spread beyond the prostate gland. With early diagnosis, anatomic nerve-sparing radical prostatectomy is possible. Of importance, even with the modification of nerve sparing at the time of radical prostatectomy, many men will experience at least a temporary deficit in their erectile function, for twelve months or more from the time of surgery. The truth is that the nerves become traumatized even with the most delicate surgical technique, and much time is required for them to heal and regain their normal function. During this time, erectile tissue in the penis may become dysfunctional and possibly remain so even after nerve function recovery occurs. For this reason, many urologists promote early sexual activity, as I do, following radical prostatectomy. The concept of "erection rehabilitation" has come to the fore lately, with concerns that highly motivated, sexually interested individuals may wish to explore alternatives to allow sexual activity following surgery to attempt to preserve erectile function as much as possible. Specialists in this field also continue to make scientific discoveries that may assist with nerve function recovery. I should also mention that prosthesis surgery can be performed without delay following the radical prostatectomy in the case of a man who has had significant erectile dysfunction before the surgery took place, or if the patient required extensive local periprostatic excision (extensive removal of tissue surrounding the prostate) for the removal of the cancer. The importance of these issues is not lost on many champions of male health, and support must continue for ongoing research work that results in preserved sexual function in all men requiring prostate cancer treatment.

PART II

Considering Options and Treatments

7

Scott Erskine and Susan Erskine

Research CSI *Style: The Importance of Being Thorough*

Scott Erskine was an FBI supervisor in charge of counterterrorism for all the hostage-taking of American citizens overseas. His cases included investigating the bombing of Pan Am flight 103 in 1988, the assassination attempt on President George H. W. Bush in Kuwait in 1993, and the bombings in Saudi Arabia in 1995 and 1996. He had responsibility for Europe, the Middle East, and Africa. Scott and his wife, Susan, live in a gracious home in the Washington, D.C., suburb of Centreville, Virginia. We sat down together in May 2006, shortly after he had retired from the FBI at age sixty, and spoke about his experience with prostate cancer and how the couple dealt with it.

Scott says it began with a message on his telephone answering machine. It was from his doctor, who apologized for having to leave a message like this: "I wanted to let you know as soon as possible that one of your [biopsy] core samples came back positive."

Scott is a distinguished-looking man with gray hair and a great sense of presence. He speaks in a quiet but firm voice. "When I heard about the diagnosis, I was a little shaken, but after that I realized it was just another challenge of life. And we approached it in a pragmatic way."

Susan seconds the statement. "He kinda buried his worries and fears and just decided to attack it as he would one of his cases." Susan, a vivacious, warm, and attractive former elementary school teacher, is a first-rate team player. "Immediately we were off to the bookstore to pick up and read everything we could find on the subject. We came back with five books, and we read all of them over the course of a week. We read together, we compared our thoughts, we underlined, we highlighted, we researched!"

Scott recalls that back in the 1980s, when he took his annual FBI physicals, his PSAs were edging up past 4.4, and at some point he became concerned and asked his general practitioner to recommend a local urologist. "He did a sonogram as well as the standard biopsy. All six of them were negative, but he found some shadowing on the sonogram. That meant an area of suspicion. I repeated the biopsy with the same urologist, and though he kept increasing the number of core samples, he still couldn't find anything. Yet my PSA kept going up and down. It never got above 10. I eventually left that urologist and went down to Georgetown University Hospital to a Dr. Reynolds, and over a three-year period he would put me to sleep and do multiple biopsies. And finally in 2001, they did find cancer in one of the last eighteen biopsy cores. I had seventy-eight [core samples] taken over a five-year period! The PSA would go down with [the antibiotic] Cipro but would always come back up. I just thought something was there. I probably had prostatitis. I had difficulty urinating but no bleeding. So I just insisted that Dr. Reynolds do this procedure every year until we found it."

Meantime, Scott continued his research. He began hearing about such favorable outcomes from friends who had been through brachytherapy (seed implants) that he began leaning in that direction. "I knew it was much less invasive than other therapies." But Susan was unconvinced and completely opposed the idea. "I'm a very controlling person, so I thought I could take over the solution to his problem. I tried to solve everybody else's problems with my own ideas, and Scott very quickly let me know that he had a handle on it, and it was *his* decision. So I relented a little bit. I was opposed to it because of what had happened to my stepfather. He had decided that he did not want to have any impotence or incontinence, so he definitely would not be going to do anything that would lead to that. He did the cryo [cryotherapy] thing—freezing the prostate. It escaped the capsule and went to his bones. In the end that was his downfall and that's what killed him. So when Scott put his foot down and said, 'I know how you feel,' I kept saying, 'I'd rather have you alive and impotent than in the ground and potent.' I had read a line and kept repeating it, 'When in doubt, get it out.' And what I was pushing for was the surgery."

Still, Scott wanted to look into brachytherapy further. Susan agreed but said, "Promise me that if we investigate every single avenue of brachytherapy thoroughly till you're satisfied, will you then look at the other option with me?" And his reply was yes. Scott continues, "So we took a trip down to the radiological labs in Georgia, just outside of Atlanta, which I'd heard about and read a lot about. They're the pioneers in the procedure of putting seeds in first and then using the seeds as targets for the external beam radiation. They've had some very good results [reported] in doing it that way. However, most of the patients who had gone through the brachytherapy were [later] impotent!" For Scott Erskine, that fact meant case closed on brachytherapy. Next stop Johns Hopkins, where he met with urologist Dr. Arthur Burnett. "He immediately had his pathology department examine my slides and he confirmed that, yes, it was cancer. He said, 'Seventy-eight biopsies . . . don't have a problem with your rectum. My boys don't leak, and you'll be fully potent after two years.' We chose Dr. Burnett and the prostatectomy on several factors. Number one, the prostate is removed. Number two, the surgeon can feel the margins to see whether cancer has spread beyond the prostate capsule. And number three, he can do a biopsy of the lymph system around the prostate.

"I knew it would be a long recovery and we decided to go along with it because I was in very good shape. I was fifty-six when I had the operation done. I didn't smoke, and therefore we thought that would provide the longest survival rate, even though we might have some immediate complications. We also knew a lot of patients have terrible problems with their bowel system and then the impotency problem after five years if they go for radiation. It destroys the good tissue as well as the bad."

And what has been the fallout for Scott? "Oh, I'm fine! They took the catheter out after two weeks. After they took it out, I leaked a little during the day, but I was dry every single night. I could walk. I could lift weights. I went back to playing tennis at the end of the fourth week. I was just very lucky. I went back to work at the end of four and a half weeks. I've had no interference with physical activity since my operation. None whatsoever. I used to run. I can't run now because of arthritis in my knees, but I play golf, I lift weights, and I walk a lot. And when it comes to sexual activities, I have to use Viagra. But otherwise, as I've said, I'm doing just fine.

"When other men ask me what the surgery was like, I tell them quite candidly that the first twenty-four hours are the most painful . . . the most discomfort. I tell them when you get nauseous, you ask for a shot; you don't ask for a pill. I tell them how after twenty-four hours every day improves exponentially.

"It's extremely important that you share everything with your partner, that he or she is part of the decision-making process so there are no surprises. It shouldn't complicate the marriage or partnership any further than it has to. My wife is very understanding. She's very thankful and we can look at each other and smile, and I can say I'm cancer-free."

It was a very difficult time for Susan. "My mother was diagnosed with Alzheimer's, and so we moved her here and I was taking care of Mom." (Scott interrupts: "And *me*!" Susan smiles and tells him, "That's so sweet. Thank you!") "To tell you the truth, I tried sharing Scott's condition with our tennis friends. We shared the news and my feeling as a woman, because I know men are very different and unemotional about things. As soon as I told my friends, I was expecting them to go, 'Oh! What can we do?' 'I'm so sorry.' On the contrary, the reaction was, 'That's nothing . . . prostate cancer is nothing . . . everybody gets it . . . you didn't have to have surgery because it's so slow-growing, it'll never kill you and . . .' It's, 'Play tennis!' There was no compassion, no sympathy, no questions asked, no care, no concern, because they were ignorant of the disease. Entirely ignorant. It was like Scott had a cold. But our male friends . . . they were different. They knew it was serious. Those that knew about prostate cancer. You know what I'd like to say to other wives whose husbands are going through the same thing? Well, the first thing is that you should learn as much as you can—be as educated as you can about all aspects of prostate cancer and its treatments and its outcomes. Secondly, be as open as you can with your spouse. If it means to set aside your fears and emotions for a while, you might have to do that. Because you're not the one, even though you're sharing the experience of the disease—ultimately it's your husband's decision. Support him—be open to changes that the diagnosis and treatment will present in your lives. And surround yourself with friends and family who will bring you some support. Because you're so busy doing for your husband—*you* need that support as well."

Following his retirement from the FBI, Scott Erskine became the executive director of the Society of Former Special Agents of the FBI, Inc., an organization dedicated to the assistance and welfare of former FBI agents and their families. They have 130 chapters nationwide and a foundation that provides $300,000 in scholarships every year as well as $200,000 in financial assistance to those former agents and their families who are in need. It's quite an operation and a full-time job.

The Doctor's Notebook

Scott Erskine's clinical case offers some important lessons. First, he and his wife, Susan, are to be commended for being so proactive after learning of Scott's diagnosis. I admire his approach toward having the disease. He saw it simply as another challenge in his life, and he was prepared to deal with it. And his manner of dealing with it was not just to be courageous while accepting the diagnosis. Rather, he went about learning about the disease and his treatment options. He did his homework! I am glad he did, and I believe he made the very best choice for himself as a relatively young, healthy man with many good years ahead of him. Another element in his story is the tremendous support of his wife. It is quite clear that Susan's abiding encouragement made a difference for him.

His story also offers lessons with regard to the management of prostate cancer. There were dilemmas associated with his diagnosis. Scott had been under the careful watch of a urologist, and I take my hat off to both him and his urologists, who were diligent in his care. His story, however, once again reflects the imprecision of PSA testing. In his case, PSA values had risen enough to give concern, prompting repeated prostate biopsy sessions. I would like to emphasize that *only a prostate biopsy, which produces tissue for the pathologist to look at, is specific in making the diagnosis.* Sometimes patients do require repeat biopsy sessions if concerns persist. Perhaps in the future we will be able to develop other less invasive although highly diagnostic procedures that would supplant the role of biopsy.

This case history also is informative with regard to expectations following radical prostatectomy as it is performed today. Scott underwent a standard "open" radical prostatectomy that involved an incision at the low part of the abdomen (retropubic surgical approach). As his testimony shows, he had a rapid recovery both in the immediate postoperative interval as well as several weeks down the line. In fact, the surgery is performed in about an hour and a half, and hospitalization stays are now only two days. Patients uniformly have a rapid return to physical activity. Urinary incontinence is usually met for most patients within several weeks following surgery, with relatively few men experiencing long-term, significant urinary incontinence. Erectile dysfunction is quite common early, although the majority of men with preoperative levels of intact erectile function who are able to undergo a nerve-sparing procedure recover erectile function. The outcomes for many are quite favorable to preserve satisfactory sexual intercourse ability. Bowel function complications are generally unheard of with a standard open retropubic technique.

All in all, his case proceeded quite well. It also reveals that the open surgical approach remains quite successful for disease eradication while preserving functional outcomes. Many patients today perceive that laparoscopic and robotic surgical approaches are superior, but this premise is incorrect. These are relatively new introductions to the technique of surgery, and their actual success rates, at least for the long term, remain to be understood. Without question, the overarching principle that all patients must consider when proceeding ahead with radical prostatectomy is to identify a highly trained, experienced surgeon who knows his outcomes and can perform the surgery well irrespective of the surgical approach.

8

Arnold Palmer

Driving Prostate Cancer Under Par

His grin is as broad as a violin bow and his demeanor as warm as Florida sunshine. He sits behind a golf course–size executive desk, enveloped by piles of papers and a plethora of family pictures. He is, after all, Arnold Palmer, the man whose very being spells golf. Beside him is his yellow lab, Mulligan, forever ready to accept a gift of nibbles.

You can hardly believe Arnold Palmer was seventy-eight when he spoke with us in early January 2008. He has remained energetic and retained his enthusiasm for life. His celebrity status has never gone to his head. "I don't think of myself as a celebrity. I just think that I'm a golfer. And a person who likes to make people happy and do things that help people, and I get a lot of satisfaction out of seeing pleasure in other people."

He was but three years old when his father, Milfred "Deacon" Palmer, a golf professional, placed a golf club in his hands and began teaching him to play. Deacon Palmer had other lessons for his son that have stayed with him. "From the day I started my father always said, 'Remember one thing. Golf is a game! Play it like a game.'" Probably the professional golfer today is taking it a little more seriously than he really should. "Also what he taught me, too, was a solid set of values. Like manners. To be polite and to treat other people like I would like to be treated." These are lessons that help reveal the foundation of his integrity and explain why those who meet him are taken with his kindness.

Arnold Palmer was born in Latrobe, Pennsylvania, on September 10, 1929. His father worked at the Latrobe Country Club as the course superintendent and provided his young son with training and encouragement. Not surprisingly, by the time Arnie, as he was affectionately known, reached his teens, he had begun defeating the older caddies. In high school, he won his first tournament, the prestigious West Penn Amateur Championship, and went on to take national junior golf championships. While a student at Wake Forest University he became one of the nation's leading collegiate players.

Arnold turned pro in 1955, winning the Canadian Open. He won the Masters Tournament four times, the U.S. Open in 1960, and the British Open in 1961 and 1962. His remarkable performance on the country's premier golf courses won him nineteen titles and some of the highest-paying prizes of the time. Before the end of 1963 he was the leading money winner and twice represented the United States in the prestigious Ryder Cup Match, in 1963 as the victorious team captain.

The Associated Press named Arnold Palmer "Athlete of the Decade" for his extraordinary effect on the game during the sixties. Accolades followed in an avalanche: the Hickok Professional Athlete of the Year and *Sports Illustrated*'s Sportsman of the Year trophies. Palmer was inducted into the World Golf Hall of Fame, the American Golf Hall of Fame, and the PGA Hall of Fame. Since his first professional victory, in 1955, to the end of 1997, he has won ninety-two championships in both national and international tournaments. His incredible performance on the greens and his immense popularity with fans drew a contingent of followers whom television sportscasters tagged "Arnie's Army." They continue to follow his golf engagements to this day.

During Arnold Palmer's hottest stretch, in the sixties, the golf champion hired a business manager, Mark McCormack, and began building an entrepreneurial network. Today, Arnold is the president of Arnold Palmer Enterprises. Many of his commercial activities are golf-oriented ventures.

At the same time, Palmer is a staunch philanthropist, helping to fund worthy causes, particularly those related to hospitals and medical research. He has helped establish the Arnold Palmer Hospital for Children in Orlando, as well as the Arnold Palmer Prostate Center at the Eisenhower Lucy Curci Cancer Center in Rancho Mirage, California, a project brought about through his close friendship with President Eisenhower. For more than twenty years, Arnold has served as the honorary national chairman of the March of Dimes Birth Defects Foundation.

Given that his days are filled with business decisions and his mind is never far from his favorite pastime, hypothetically, how would Arnold Palmer ever choose between the two? A pure Solomon's choice. "Well, you can't ignore certainly the entrepreneurial aspects of the game because they're evident; they're obvious. But, at the same time, it's equally if not more important than the entrepreneurial aspects. And playing it, like my father always said, playing it as a game. Don't ever forget that.

"And the caliber of the golfer has changed in that the golfer that played the tour when I started playing fifty-five years ago was a golf professional in the sense that his main business was teaching and running country clubs. Today, in this modern world, that person has now become a professional golfer. A professional golfer is the guy who plays golf for a living. And a golf professional works at teaching and running country clubs—that sort of thing."

It is clear that Arnold Palmer attributes his many accomplishments, both professionally and personally, to the close relationship he had with his father and the respect he had for him. "One of the proudest moments for me," he says, "was when I convinced my dad that I was a professional golfer." He also takes great pride in being able to establish the Winnie Palmer Hospital for Women and Babies, named in honor of his late wife, and the Latrobe Area Hospital Charitable Foundation where he grew up in Latrobe, Pennsylvania.

Arnold's own brush with prostate cancer led him to become an advocate for the eradication of the disease. He is very open in telling how he dealt with the cancer and in giving advice to those who are today struggling with it. "A lot of people don't like to talk about prostate cancer because they don't want to think about something that could or may end their lives. Or something they might have to endure. Let me tell you, when I was a young man and went to school, I had a good friend who graduated from school and went on to college, and then went to medical school. That man became my doctor. And he was not only a friend, but he was one of the highest-ranking and thought-of physicians in my town. And he was my doctor. I have to say that I am alive today because of that man and the fact that I had a physical every year!

"And, of course, that goes with a lot of people. A lot of people do what I did. A lot of people do not do what I did. And the ones that do not are at risk! They are at risk because what could be caught at a very early age becomes at some stage a death penalty. The people who do go and have a physical are able to talk to a physician and explain to that physician what might be bothering them and that could lead to an early discovery of prostate cancer. I am today involved in prostate cancer largely because I myself went through—whatever you want to call it—this ordeal. And that's what led me to get involved in helping set up the Arnold Palmer Prostate Center in Palm Springs.

"In my case, I had the physicals, and of course as various new things came to the surface my doctor would tell me that there was a new procedure. I was forty at the time. And when he told me about these things, one of these things turned out to be the PSA. And I had no idea what he was talking about. And he asked me if he could do my PSA, and I certainly gave him my permission. Well, in the years coming on, he checked my PSA every year. And it remained in tolerance. It started out at 1, went to 2, and after years later, went to 3, and in more recent years went to 4! And when it went to 4, my doctor said, 'We're gonna watch you closely. Maybe,' he said, 'we'll do it every six months.' And he did. One year in that six-month period, it went to 4.2. And he called me and said, 'Arnie, we really have to look into doing biopsies of your prostate,' so the next few years we did the biopsies. And he followed it very closely. Negative. Negative. Then one year it was positive.

"That was 1996, and that was twelve years ago. I was sixty-six. I had cancer! They had done six [cores] in each biopsy session. And the last one made eighteen biopsies. Just one or two showed positive. One thing they didn't do in the beginning was enough biopsy cores! In other words, six biopsy cores does not cover the range of the prostate that should be covered.

"The standard today, I believe, is fourteen, but that was earlier. By the time they had taken eighteen biopsies, which was [over] three years, they discovered that I had prostate cancer. Well, when I went above 4 [PSA] and went to 5 and onward, that should have been more of an indication that there was cancer, but the biopsies were not hitting the right spots!

"Soon as my doctor determined I had cancer throughout the biopsies, of course, I was as concerned as anybody would be, and I turned to my doctor and said, 'Where do I go, Bob?' And he said, 'Let me look into that.' And he did.

"My doctor did all the research for me. He was a very caring and thorough man, and remember, he was my good friend. That of course helped. Before I chose surgery, he gave me all the other options. Whether radiation or whatever . . . and I made my choice with his help. I asked him what he thought, and we discussed the various options. In any event, he said, 'There are several places you can go. You can go to Johns Hopkins. You can go to the Mayo Clinic . . .' And I said—out of the blue—'Let's just go to the Mayo Clinic.' I guess because I knew some doctors there, so I made that decision to go to the Mayo. This was on a Friday night. I got into my airplane and flew to Orlando, picked up my wife and daughter, and we all flew out to Rochester, Minnesota. That Sunday night I checked in. I have to say I felt confident that everything was gonna work out. Yep! I was confident. Because I wasn't smart enough to know anything different. What I knew was that I was in the care of the right people and I had the confidence in what they would do.

"Of course, I did ask questions about the possible outcomes of the operation [the possibilities of incontinence and potency problems], and it was all explained to me . . . and I was happy to hear what they were telling me. And that they were going to try to do nerve sparing.

"You want to know how it all worked out? I'll tell you. Certainly." He was smiling now. "I'm a happy guy. It works! And as for the incontinence, I would have to say that if you have a radical, you know that for six weeks or so you're gonna be under.

I had my operation on Tuesday, and I came home on Friday. For six weeks I did the normal things. You know, you have the catheter. I had the whole thing. So after six weeks I was free to go! If I remember right, I was dry after that. And I was back on the golf course in six weeks. Period!

"My PSA was zero. And I've had one every six months after that. And it remains at zero. And that was ten years ago!

"Do you know that I have on average five phone calls a week—and letters—asking me about prostate cancer! Men asking me what they should do about prostate cancer. Well, I'm not a doctor. But I can tell them my experience. And then when I do that, my recommendation is, of course, their choice. My doctor gave me my choice. I would say to you—if you told me you had prostate cancer and you asked me what to do, I would say you have options. And those options improve every day. I don't mind telling you that I had a radical. It is now ten years past my operation and I feel like a newly married young man! And that is the happiest thing I can tell you.

"What I would say to somebody who has the misfortune of having advanced cancer? I would say that you must sit down with your doctor and seek the best advice he or she can give. I can tell that person that they can go to the Arnold Palmer Prostate Center in Palm Springs, California. They can go to Johns Hopkins. To the Mayo Clinic. To any major cancer center where they have great research in the realm of prostate cancer. If they have a PSA of 10 or more, they must be under constant observation. But a high number like that does not mean it's all over. It just means you have to be more concerned and closely observed.

"In my own case, my wife, Winnie, was a gem. She was very supportive and never backed off. The unfortunate thing in my life is that she became a cancer patient herself shortly after I did. And she did not have the good fortune to have had the knowledge or medical expertise to be able to do something about her own situation. I took her to every major cancer center in the United States, and we did everything humanly possible through medicine to cure her. Unfortunately, the cancer had gone too far and it was too late to save her. Early discovery and early treatment is probably the most important single thing I can tell anybody about any cancer."

The Doctor's Notebook

From Arnold Palmer's account, it is quite evident that he is a happy man. He provides the outlook of a man who has conquered prostate cancer and eliminated it from worry. His charmed life did not occur by accident. It resulted from early guidance about how to live life in a joyful way and by building supportive relationships. He is one to take on life's challenges with zealous determination and a winning attitude. His sources of support have come from many, from his father to his wife, and even his special army. He built a strong relationship with his personal physician, and accordingly he benefited from early diagnosis and treatment of his prostate cancer.

Arnold speaks of some of the dilemmas of early diagnosis. Indeed, the urologist's diagnostic armamentarium is not perfect. Our current diagnostic tools, including PSA testing, digital rectal examination, and prostate ultrasound procedures with biopsy of the prostate, are definite improvements over the prior era in the management of this disease. Applying these tools, we have been able to make earlier and better diagnoses of prostate cancer, resulting in many lives being saved. But Arnold's case history reveals that these tools still remain inexact. Elevated PSA measurements do not always mean prostate cancer. Multiple biopsy sessions sometimes are required before a prostate cancer diagnosis can be firmly made by a pathologist looking at the biopsied prostate tissue under a microscope. In recent years, biopsy instruments have been better developed to be better tolerated, allowing twelve or more biopsy cores to be taken (unlike in the past when only six cores or less could be tolerated). With more biopsy cores that can be obtained, a better sampling of the prostate can be done, and a more accurate determination of the current condition may result. Efforts will continue to refine our diagnostic tools to make the diagnosis of prostate cancer early, efficiently, and noninvasively. Improvements in prostate cancer diagnosis will make many winners out of men who are or will become afflicted by this disease.

9

Robin Cole

A Celebrated Linebacker's Charge to the End Zone

Robin Cole is a former professional All-Pro linebacker for the Pittsburgh Steelers and the New York Jets. During his twelve-year football career, he played in Super Bowls XIII and XIV and established himself among his peers as one of the very best linebackers in football. He occupies an honored place in the All Western Athletic Conference for former top players. At the age of forty-eight, Robin Cole faced his toughest opponent when he was diagnosed with prostate cancer. We spoke with him in January 2008, when he was fifty-three. This is his story.

"I grew up and went to school in Compton, California, a suburb of Los Angeles. I come from a rather large middle-class African American family. I'm one of ten siblings—I'm number seven. I have seven brothers and two sisters. My father was a body fender repairman. My mother was a home cleaner and housekeeper for doctor friends of ours, and today both of our families are very, very close. My high school years were fantastic years. I developed really nice relationships there, and, thanks to the Internet, we're still able to keep up with one another today. Throughout high school I played some baseball, wrestled, and then got to play football. I became really good at my sport, and from that point

I had the opportunity to go to college. I spent from 1973 to 1977 at the University of New Mexico, and that's where I became All-American. Then in 1977 I was drafted by the Pittsburgh Steelers in the first round. That was my vision—a dream of mine—something that once I got out of college became a reality. I owe so much of my success to the people around me—the people who encouraged me and believed in me maybe more than I believed in myself back then. And I knew that I had a pretty strong work ethic, and because of that work ethic I think I was able just to stay focused, continue to work hard, and tell myself that the doors will eventually open for me—and they *did*!"

Throughout his career with Pittsburgh, television sportscasters called Robin Cole—number 56—the one solid team player the Steelers could always count on. Today, you will find his name in the New Mexico Hall of Fame and in the Albuquerque Hall of Fame, and he is a sports celebrity at his alma mater, the University of New Mexico.

"We can think about all those great moments, but you have to realize that it takes a journey to get you there. Because if you think about it, that great moment is but a flash. Bingo! It's gone! You remember those moments, but I really found out, as I got older, that the journey is what you really have to enjoy. The journey of getting there, that's the thing you're gonna live with. That's what's gonna be with you forever, and it's the thing that's gonna take you further ahead than any one event. But there are some events along the way that are really crucial to getting there—the highlights. One of biggest ones was, I was in a game, and after the game was over, I realized that I was the MVP pick, all the way up to the fourth quarter. Now, nothing changed me in the fourth quarter. I continued to play well. But in that fourth quarter a guy by the name of Terry Bradshaw threw a couple of bombs that put us ahead in that game. *He* ended up as the MVP!" Robin laughs. "And that was Super Bowl XIV, where I had the opportunity to play back home in Pasadena, California. That was just twenty-five miles from my house, and we played the Los Angeles Rams in front of my home crowd, family, and friends, and that was one of the highlights, and then to be able to put on a show in that game!"

In 1988, when Pittsburgh cut him after more than a decade, Robin Cole joined the New York Jets. In one game, the Jets had just been routed 28–3 by the New England Patriots. Cole became an instant leader. He rallied his new teammates: "We won't let the Steelers intimidate us. It's just a matter of stopping them before they stop us. We're gonna do this and we're gonna make it work." And they did. It was a 24–20 victory over the Steelers. Jets coach Joe Walton said of Cole, "He's smart. He played with a great organization and played in two Super Bowls. But he's also good people. He knows how this game should be played and how you should act. The key thing about Robin is the class he adds to the team."

Robin continues, "I'm a God-fearing man. I believe in faith, and faith moves mountains. Because of my faith I think there's a series of reasons why every now and then when I get knocked down I just seem to get right back up, and I guess I'll be that way until my last day. So from there, I'm back here in the Pittsburgh area. My wife is a nurse, and we have four kids. Our oldest son has a Ph.D. in computer and information systems in a college down in Memphis. Our second son is at Chapel Hill finishing a master's degree as a strength and conditioning coach at the University of North Carolina. I've got two daughters, one a sophomore in college at a Jesuit university in Wheeling, West Virginia. The other is graduating from high school. Both of them want to be teachers.

"I was thirty-three years old when I found I had to leave football. I had my share of injuries, including a dislocated toe. And when I told them I needed surgery, they decided to cut me, so they fired me! That was the National Football League in those days—that was 1988. You know, players don't get a chance to say, 'Hey, I've had enough.' You know, you have an injury, you get older, they do what they did to me—the league just drops you. They don't give you the opportunity to take a year off and heal up and get well. I wasn't old and I played twelve years. That's a lot for a linebacker."

Robin has always tried to stay in top physical condition. He has had annual physicals over the years ever since his high school days. When he began playing professional football he says doctors began keeping tabs on his prostate, making sure he had no problems. He says he was only in his twenties when he got his first DRE exam. "I was pretty much zero. My [PSA] numbers remained pretty much zero all the way up until I think two years prior to their starting to climb up to 1. Then they started moving a little bit. From 1 to 2. That happened within a year. And when it moved to 2, we thought we needed to take it a little further because at that time two of my brothers were already diagnosed with prostate cancer. I was now forty-eight."

What was happening to Robin, he began to realize, was rapidly becoming a family affair. "My first brother was right around the same age as I was when his PSAs started to move up, too. My youngest brother was forty when his began to rise to three-point-something. My father never told us what his PSA was. And he never told us he was having challenges. His challenge in his late thirties turned out to be urine. He had to use the restroom all the time. That was a sign. We never knew then, and he never shared with us that he was having his challenge. He was walking around and didn't know that he had prostate cancer. We knew things were bothering him, but he never would take it further. Finally, he went to the doctor, and only because somebody asked him to go, but still he wouldn't share any information with us. We learned later that his cancer had metastasized and was in his lungs. Then five years later it was in his other lung—it had spread. He went to the VA hospital and they couldn't remove the second lung so they closed him up and he lived as long as he could. At the age of forty-nine he passed away—we thought of lung cancer! Little did we know that my father's death was actually caused by prostate cancer. The mystery of his death didn't begin to unravel until one of my older brothers was diagnosed with prostate cancer."

Gradually, Robin began to connect the dots after a second older brother was diagnosed three years later, followed by Robin's two younger brothers. Both had surgery and are alive today. But Cole's father was one of thirteen siblings. Two of his brothers had died, and Robin immediately began to suspect that the cause of his uncles' deaths had been prostate cancer. Robin immediately set out to warn his cousins to get checked. When Robin's own PSA passed 2, his primary physician sent him to a urologist. The year was 2004. "My wife, who is an OR [operating room] nurse, made sure I went to a good urologist. The urologist said, 'We can watch this—or we can find out for sure what's going on.' I told him I want to know. So first he did the rectal exam and said he didn't feel anything. 'You're smooth,' he said. 'There's nothing there. I'm ready to believe there's nothing there.' But I told him I want to know, so he says, 'Okay, let's do the biopsy.' It came back and my prostate was twenty-five percent cancerous. He said he couldn't believe it because he didn't see any sign of it from the DRE. But he did acknowledge that the PSA is very important. That rectal is important, too, he said, but those PSA numbers told us something *could* be happening. It may not always be cancer but [in this case] something is happening.

"When the doctor spoke to me, he was pretty sensitive. He understood about my brothers and he sat down and gave me options. He said, 'Go home and talk to your wife and decide what you guys wanna do.' He told me I would probably be best having the surgery, but he himself didn't do it. He said, 'If you were in your sixties I would say, try the seeds, or try radiation, those kinds of things. But because you're so young, you're probably gonna want the surgery—you probably will wanna have it out.'

"My wife says, 'Robin, you're forty-eight years old. It's best to get it all out.' All along *I* was thinking of the radical prostatectomy. Two of my brothers had had it and they were doing well. But my wife says, 'The doctors around here have been talking about this new surgery that's out. It's called laparoscopic.' But she says, 'Nobody around here does it. I do know though that it's available somewhere.' So she says she's gonna get on the Internet and find out who does it. She told me she's starting to do the research, and then I started reading about prostate cancer, too.

"Because of my insurance, I had to go for a second opinion. I found out that if I wanted to get this particular procedure [laparoscopic surgery], I would have to go outside of network. So I went to see a Dr. Sanders, who was the head of the urology department at the major teaching hospital in Pittsburgh. He had trained under Dr. [Patrick] Walsh, who was the head of urology at Johns Hopkins. And Dr. Sanders gave me a copy of Dr. Walsh's book called *Dr. Patrick Walsh's Guide to Surviving Prostate Cancer*. I read the whole book. And in the book, Dr. Walsh is talking about laparoscopic surgery. He had some negative things to say about it. Like it wasn't proven and blah, blah, blah. He probably wrote the book when the laparoscopic prostatectomy was just getting started. Because now I understand they teach it at quite a few medical schools. And a guy I learned to trust spoke highly of the procedure. Then my wife found the Web site of a surgeon in Florida who developed an expertise in laparoscopic surgery. And after she studied the information on the site, she got excited and suggested I contact that doctor.

"She went on to explain first how a radical prostatectomy was done. She says, 'You're gonna be down for about six to eight weeks, you know. The doctor can't really see your prostate. He has to feel it. Okay?' And she says in a lot of cases there's a lot of tissue that's unnecessarily taken from the body that doesn't need to be removed. Then she talked about the newer technique. The way they explain it, she says, it's similar to the laparoscopic gallbladder procedure, where they go in and pump it with air, and the doctor can see with a camera what he's working on, which is something in that other technique [the radical open prostatectomy] he couldn't do.

"Anyhow, I called this doctor up and made an appointment to go down and see him. When we sat down to talk, I said, 'Golly, doc, if you can see what's going on inside me, I think that's a whole lot better.' But I already had made up my mind. I was gonna elect to do the other technique—the open radical one—because in that procedure they can do that nerve-sparing technique. That's when he explains to me, 'I can do the same technique. There's no differ-ence.' He says, 'I can feel what I'm cutting—everything's attached to that.' And he convinced me laparoscopic was the way I would go. And that was that!

"What appealed to me about the laparoscopic surgery was that three of my brothers had the other technique [open radical prostatectomy], and they were down. And if I can have the same results without cutting me open—because I already have six scars on me—that's what I'm trying to avoid. This surgeon knew about nerve sparing. If I were gonna do the [open] radical, I would have gone to a doctor who knows how to do that. Some doctors do it and some don't. But the key here was this: the surgeon could see inside with the camera. And I said if he's gonna do a nerve-sparing technique—if he can *see* what he's doing, what nerves he's sparing, and touching—that was the key with me."

Did Robin's surgeon explain that one major criticism of the laparoscopic procedure is that there are no long-term studies supporting the claim that the benefits of laparoscopy outweigh those of the open radical procedure?

"Oh yeah. So maybe there were no long-term studies in the United States yet. There *were* long-term studies in Europe, the surgeon says. Because they had been doing the technique prior—quite a few years, the surgeon tells me, in Europe. That's where he trained. One of the things is that there were less challenges with incontinence. The numbers of positive results [from laparoscopy] were higher. And there are also, as far as the erection is concerned, there was more success. My own outcome is good, but still, I think I still need some help down there, I think maybe a lot of it is partly mental.

"My outcomes have been good. Shortly after the operation I would have to wear four or five pads [to deal with the incontinence]. That lasted a few months. The only challenge I had, if I was working out or straining. If I wasn't doing anything straining, I wouldn't have any problems. When I started playing golf, a little strain, well, then I'd leak a little bit, but I would say that I was dry within six months. I was on the golf course in about six months. Nowhere can you expect [better] with a major surgery like that. You're eliminating the key muscles that would stop your urinating. But now I have no problems and my PSAs have been excellent."

Robin says his surgeon was careful to point out that being certain that cancer will never return always represents a challenge for the doctor. No one can offer a guarantee. Does that thought disturb Robin Cole?

"No, it doesn't. Because, look—it's like with an automobile. You gotta come back and get it repaired again. Same thing with laparoscopic surgery. But so far, nobody's been back! Everybody I know that's had this procedure, it's been fantastic. I have a younger brother who had it done at UCLA—he's doing fine. My laparoscopic surgeon has done hundreds of these procedures. He's busy all the time."

Meantime, upon reflection, Robin will confess that besides his passion for football, he has always had a passion for food, which accounts for his present occupation. He has taken off his jersey and helmet and substituted them with a baker's hat and apron. Today, he runs Robin Cole's Gourmet Cheesecakes in Pittsburgh. His inspiration came from his grandmother, who ran a restaurant and her own bakery. "She made the most phenomenal hamburgers. I have never had a sweet potato pie that tastes like hers or a peach or apple cobbler that tasted like hers. And, oh, her German chocolate cake was just a bomb. I knew way back then that someday I would be in the food business—and here I am."

Robin Cole's scrimmage with prostate cancer has also led him to become involved in helping men and their families deal with the disease. He has established a prostate cancer foundation in Pittsburgh to promote education, awareness, and early detection as well as to lend support to prostate cancer patients. (See the Obediah Cole Foundation in the resources section.)

Surviving cancer, Robin says, is all about hope. "That hope has to come from within you. Really, it does. When a person says he has no hope, you have to remind him, 'Brother, you need a dream.' He may ask you, 'Where do I get a dream from?' You give him a dream . . . something to go after, something he can put his hands on, touch it, make a difference in the lives of other people or the community. All of a sudden that's where he gets hope from. You gotta give a guy a dream. A person can't quit on himself. Once a person quits on himself, when he gives up, that's when the hope is gone. All hope is not gone until you are no longer there! We must tell these people, 'We'd like you to be around. We'd like you to see your grandchildren. Don't let a disease that's curable— one hundred percent curable if it's detected early enough—knock you out of the game. We want you in the game!'"

The Doctor's Notebook

Family is a word that leaps to mind after absorbing Robin Cole's story. He comes from a big family with many brothers. Quite obviously, they have all stayed very well connected even into adulthood, and with their close contact and mutual support he was familiar with the reality of prostate cancer. With his father dying at a young age and many brothers found to carry prostate cancer, it was all but certain that he too would be diagnosed with it. His family exemplifies the hereditary basis of many forms of prostate cancer. The lesson here is that if you have a brother or father who has had prostate cancer, your risk of having this disease is heightened. Being proactive about getting tested for it, particularly with this observation of risk, as Robin did, may well be the most important action for any individual to take to defeat prostate cancer.

Robin's case history provides an opportunity to review several talking points about the laparoscopic innovation to prostate cancer surgery. The laparoscopic approach represents an alternative way to perform the surgery in which several small incisions are done in the abdomen instead of a single larger one. Quite evidently, Robin was pleased to have undergone this surgical approach. At the same time, his brothers had undergone the more conventional open approach with high success as well. He emphasizes that the laparoscopic approach affords a better way to visualize surgical structures, which suggests that the surgery could be carried out better than techniques in which visualization is difficult. Fortunately, the surgery is done with a high level of visualization by *all* surgical techniques. Surgeons who have performed the surgery in the conventional way with high standards have achieved excellent surgical outcomes as well. The key point is that a properly performed surgery with any surgical approach achieves excellent outcomes. By corollary, a poorly executed surgery, such as that performed by a less than expert surgeon, irrespective of his or her surgical approach, can be expected to yield suboptimal results. It must be further emphasized that no surgical approach can automatically be considered to produce early continence and erectile function recovery for any man, as if it were a guarantee. It is good to have new approaches to carry out the surgery, including laparoscopic and robotic approaches, but be aware that these do not inherently establish better surgical outcomes.

10

Ken Griffey Sr.

A Hall of Famer Knocks the "Big One" Out of the Park

Ken Griffey Sr., now fifty-eight, is a former Major League Baseball star. He is the father of the great outfielder Ken Griffey Jr. and onetime minor leaguer Craig Griffey. Ken Sr. was first introduced to Major League Baseball in August 1973 when he joined the Cincinnati Reds. "That was my proudest moment, getting called up to the majors, because I had worked so hard and so long in the minor leagues." Ken's active career spanned over thirty years, and he was considered a prime piston in what came to be known as Cincinnati's Big Red Machine. He participated in the team's three World Series championships, in 1975, 1976, and 1990. In 2004, Ken was inducted into the Cincinnati Reds Hall of Fame.

After the 1981 season with the Reds, Ken was sent to the New York Yankees, where he played until 1986 as a utility player at first base and outfield. Injuries plagued him, and he was traded midseason to the Atlanta Braves, where he played for only one full season. He was then traded back to Cincinnati in mid-1988. In 1990, after the Reds' third championship, he was traded to the Seattle Mariners. In nearly three thousand games, Ken compiled a lifetime batting average of .296, with

152 home runs and 859 RBIs. He was also the Most Valuable Player of the 1980 All-Star Game.

Ken Griffey's son Ken Jr. joined the Seattle Mariners in 1989. On August 29, 1990, when the Cincinnati Reds released Ken Sr., he signed with the Mariners. On that date, for the first time in the history of Major League Baseball, a father and son appeared on the same team in the same game. Ken Sr. recalls what he refers to as the greatest moment in his career: the Mariners versus the Kansas City Royals. He says there he was out in left field and next to him in center field was his son Ken Jr. The Griffey duo made history again on September 14, 1990. "Junior and I then managed to homer back-to-back runs in the same game—against the Kansas City Royals. We still talk and josh each other about it. Junior tells me that he hit the ball faster, but then I come back and remind him that I hit the ball further." Fans still call them the greatest father-son team in baseball history.

A devastating car crash forced Ken Sr. out as a player in 1991. He was only forty-one. "I had a bulging disc in my neck and it fused in my neck. I couldn't turn my head to the right, and they had to put a cadaver bone in there. But that meant I was done playing baseball. Out there at the end of the '91 season, right in the middle of spring training, first year I was out in Arizona. You know, people don't understand—so many times injuries force players to retire when they're young. In baseball, football, any sport. If you have a career that spans fifteen to twenty years, you're probably gonna have to retire anywhere between thirty-five and forty."

After he left the Mariners, Ken became a roving hitting instructor in the minor leagues. "I started teaching kids how to hit. I did that, matter of fact, in the Mariner system. I'd stay five or six days at each place, and the Mariners would take care of all my expenses." Baseball runs through Ken Griffey's blood. Retirement to him is just a word, not an exercise to carry out. "What I do now is scout for the Cincinnati Reds. Retirement is really not retirement. I enjoy scouting. It gives me a chance to watch the younger kids play just about every day. And I sit at the ballpark and watch and grade 'em as I see 'em—and get paid to do it."

Ken will tell you how excited he was training his son Ken Jr. to follow in his footsteps. "He had the physical tools, but it was the mental tools that I worked on for him. There were so many things that I knew that I didn't have when I started that I wanted to pass on. I didn't know how to hit! And I had to teach myself the basic swing. Where is the best place to hit a ball? Pitchers try to keep you off balance with sliders, curveballs, so they can put you out. We didn't have roving instructors to come down like they do now and try to help these kids progress and get to the big leagues. You either hit or you were gone. I was able to make Junior understand what he needed to do in order to hit better. He's a natural. His eye-to-hand coordination was probably the best I'd ever seen for a kid! When he got to be fourteen and I couldn't strike him out, that's when I knew he was real good. He used to try to emulate me. And that was being crouched over and stuff. And all of a sudden, he started standing straight up because he knew he had a little more power. And that's how he developed that little wiggle that he has. And he went on and did his own thing. Dick Williams, the manager in Seattle, saw Junior at seventeen and said, 'Why can't we put him on the team right now? He's the only one who can run, hit, catch, and throw in this club.'"

Ken loves to reminisce about some of the big moments in his career, such as the time he got to play first base with the New York Yankees. "I would have to say next would be the opportunity to play my first full year in the leagues when Cincinnati went on to win the world championship in '75. They said it was one of the best series ever played, and I played well in that series. Then in 1980, in the Major League All-Star Game, when I was named MVP. But I'd have to say the most important was the opportunity to play with my son Junior."

Sometime early in 2007, Ken was faced with a major family crisis. His former wife, Alberta "Bertie" Griffey, was diagnosed with colon cancer. They had been divorced for about six years; still, he says, they remained close. (Griffey currently lives with his second wife, Val, in Winter Garden, a suburb of Orlando.) Shortly thereafter, Ken himself began developing symptoms that unnerved him. He found himself having to urinate so frequently that he decided to see his internist to find out what was going on.

"I had six uncles and they all died of prostate cancer. They were all older gentlemen and they all passed from prostate cancer. So I knew prostate cancer was prevalent in my family.

"My primary doctor in Cincinnati found that I had a PSA of 1.9. He wanted to keep an eye on me. When I went back six months later, my PSA jumped from 1.9 to almost 8.5 or 9! It was real quick. I was just trying to keep my sanity. When I told my physician about my family history, he immediately ordered a biopsy. He sent me to a urologist, a friend of his, at Christ Hospital. This urologist found that the prostate tissues were irregular. He'd done eleven cores and discovered that the cells in at least four or five of them were what he called a little strange in appearance. He never gave me a Gleason number.

"I decided to get a second opinion and I got one in Detroit. My primary sent all the slides and stuff to the doctor in Detroit, and when *he* looked at them, he agreed with the first urologist's findings. He said the cancer was not aggressive. So I went back to Cincinnati and waited another six months. My primary doctor took another biopsy and the cells looked about the same. This was about April of '07. Then around July or August they did a third biopsy, and this time they found the cells had got more aggressive and were starting to move to the other side of the prostate. That's when both doctors—my primary and my first urologist in Cincinnati—told me we'd better go ahead and get it out. The urologist was a surgeon, but he said he didn't do robotics, and I knew that was the latest. He was pushing for surgery because he said although seeds was an option, he felt that I was too young for that. Both of my doctors told me that guys who get seeds are usually around sixty-five to seventy or maybe seventy-five to eighty, and that I had a long way before I got to be that age. So they said the best thing might be to just get the prostate out. They said I could have the surgery either way—open radical or robotic.

"Junior had always been close to his mother. When he found out that Bertie had cancer and that I did too, he was pretty shaken. It kinda knocked him off his pace. First thing I did when I found out that I had prostate cancer was to call him to reassure him. He was devastated about his mom, but I told him that *I* would be okay. My cancer was not life-threatening. I said it could be taken care of quickly. Truth is, I was really worried about Junior. And I didn't want everything that was happening to affect his game. I was concerned about injuries he was having. If you're not 'there' [staying focused], you can get hurt. It's tough to hit a ball when a guy's throwing a ball ninety-eight miles an hour—sliders and curves to strike you out. You gotta face eight guys out there and the catcher, and you have the umpire, and you have to face them all by yourself. Man, it's tough. I keep telling people baseball is ninety-eight percent mental. You know, at the same time, I was also pretty worried about my other kids, my younger son, Craig, and my daughter. I mean, it was a tough time for all of us.

"There's this friend of mine who had his prostate surgery done by a doctor down in Florida who is skilled in laparoscopic surgery. He convinced me to go down there and see him, and so I took his advice. And this doc said, 'Young as you are, the best thing you can do is to have your prostate taken out.' Then he explained the ins and outs of this operation. And I thought about it and I decided to do it. That was July 10 in '07."

Ken describes his experience with laparoscopic surgery: "Right before the operation they stuck little things in my hips, in the sides of my stomach. They cut up right under your belly button. That's where they pop the prostate out. I was out cold. Only thing I remember is the catheter. Matter of fact, it's the one thing I'll never forget. I had that in almost eighteen days. And that was horrible. And the funny part was the operation was a day before 'Zo—Alonzo Mourning, the basketball player for the Miami Heat—had a big benefit golf tournament. It was a big weekend that supports inner-city kids. I was supposed to be at the golf tournament a couple of days after surgery! And I went to Miami and stood out there on the golf course for two hours and signed autographs. I felt it later, but I didn't play golf. It was enjoyable, though. I just sat there and signed autographs.

"I did have incontinence, though. It's been about five months since the surgery, but it's slowed down, and right now it's very, very little. I was wearing like three or four pads a day. I still wear pads as security just to make sure nothing happens. Now it's not as much. Every once in a while you don't have control—you gotta go to the bathroom. But, you know, the surprising thing is I go about the same like before the surgery. At night I'd go one or two times, the same as now. I'll go one or two times. Sometimes it's only one time or not at all."

Ken underscores the point that no matter which form of surgery a patient elects—open radical or laparoscopic—the ability to have full natural erections is not immediate. Traumatized spared-nerve bundles require time to recover. "The doctor tells me my erections will come back. He says he would rather have me go through all the changes—the incontinence and all that—and to make sure everything is properly healed. My wife isn't that stressed out. She's pretty good. But me? It's like you lose all your manhood. You know, I don't get ornery, mean, or anything of that nature. I will worry about it. My approach to a lot of stuff, even when I played ball, is there's a reason why certain things happen and you have to handle them in a certain way. And, like I said, I went through things with cancer and I know I'm having the erectile dysfunction process. I'm going through all that. It's not me. It's not my fault that I'm going through all of this. It's just the nature of things. If it comes, it comes. If it doesn't, it doesn't. But at the same time, you think about it. I'm worried about how my wife is gonna be. You know . . . I'm worried about how things are gonna change or whatever. And all these things are going through your head all the time. My wife is more understanding about all this than I am. It's happening to *me*, but she understands it will come back. She was telling me it could take up to a year or two. I guess she looked that up, too.

"When I go into the locker room now, and if I'm going in as a coach or into the fantasy camps now, if I were to take off my clothes and I had these pads, they'd look at you real strange. That's because they can't relate to you. They can't. So I have to be very careful how I dress, and undress, when I'm in the locker room, you know. I just walk off privately and go into a bathroom stall and do what I have to do."

How has Ken Griffey learned to cope with all the frustrations in his life? "What do I do? I take it one day at a time. I've had a lot of friends that kinda went through the same thing. They've had prostate cancer. I am able to talk to them. They actually supported *me* because they went through it before I went through it.

We might be talking about the pump and how it's supposed to be used [for erections]. I play golf with another friend of mine who uses injections. And I've recently heard from yet another about the penile implant that's supposed to work good. Meantime, my doctor says eventually the erections will come back. Another friend of mine said it took him a year. But he didn't have the robotics.

"I would like to say this: if you're a young man and you get diagnosed with prostate cancer, and if you have kids, wouldn't you rather be around for a long time and make sure they grow up and understand what life is all about? That you're telling them what's right from wrong instead of somebody else out on the street telling them? Because if you die early, you don't know what's gonna happen to them. If you find out you have prostate cancer, you want to be around for your kids. And that's basically what I think about. I have fourteen grandkids, and I want to be able to see them grow up. The youngest one is one year old. And I want to be able to see him for the next fifteen years at least and be able to see him grow up and grow up right!"

What has Ken Griffey learned from his experience fighting prostate cancer that he would like others to know? Patience, he says, is the most important word you have to understand. "With me, it's always been patience. It's allowed me to do all the things I was able to accomplish as a major-league ballplayer. As well as all the things I have ever been able to do. I'm thinking now about manhood. I may be a little worried about losing my manhood, but at the same time I still have my life! And I'm able to smile and talk to my grandkids. Talk to 'em, the boys, make sure they understand when they grow up that they know about the prostate. If you die, you're not gonna worry about manhood. 'Specially if you die young. And I'm fifty-eight—that's young. Like I say, I want to live and be able to see my grandkids grow up, know right from wrong, and be successful."

The Doctor's Notebook

Ken Griffey Sr. is proud in all the right places. He describes the effect of cancer diagnoses in his family, including his own and that of his former wife. His own prostate cancer diagnosis was important, but he put it all in the proper perspective. His perspective is that of moving ahead to deal with it but not dwelling on it in any sort of self-centered way. As with lots of other men encountering this disease, the issue of manhood is a mental challenge. I have seen many of my own patients wrestle with this dilemma, which is associated with the possibility of lost erections, even permanently, with any sort of prostate cancer treatment. One of my patients stated that he understood the risks of prostate cancer treatment, but also cleverly put this into perspective. After contending with the idea of proceeding with a radical prostatectomy, he came to realize that "the ultimate form of erectile dysfunction is death." He decided to move ahead with the surgery, which was performed expertly, and he recovered erections after all! The key message, as Ken emphasized, is that having one's life is most important, even if "manhood" is compromised. As Ken Griffey Sr. epitomizes, a proud man is one who values his life and chooses to be there for his family.

Prescriptive Information

About Radiation

The word "cure" is defined in the dictionary in a healing sense as "restoring a sick person to health." The dictionary also defines the word as a "successful treatment that brings about recovery from an illness." We mention this because there is a disagreement and an important distinction made among surgeons and radiation oncologists over what the word "cure" implies when referring to the treatment of prostate cancer.

By and large, surgeons believe that "cured" means the cancer is gone forever. Period. They further believe that if they can successfully remove the prostate and the cancer cells have not spread beyond the capsule, that ends the threat of a future recurrence of the disease, and therefore the surgical procedure can effect a "cure." The absolute end of the cancer! Consequently, the phrase "gold standard" has long been applied to surgery as it infers the best chances for a cure.

In more recent times, radiation oncologists have chosen to use the word "cure" in the belief that using today's most sophisticated technology and equipment can eliminate prostate cancer. Experienced surgeons contend, however, that with enough time radiation patients can be expected to experience a recurrence of the cancer. They would prefer that radiation oncologists speak not of "cure" but of "controlling the disease," so as to be more precise when describing radiation success. It is likely that this interdisciplinary controversy will persist until it is settled in the future by evidence-based clinical trials. Still, we think readers should be aware how the word "cure" is used and construed today.

Indeed, surgery may not be for everybody. Many men shun the very idea for any number of reasons, personal preference and lifestyle among them. A lot of men in their seventies believe that radiation represents an excellent course of treatment if they suspect that their disease may be slow-growing and not a death sentence. Some young men speak of "not wanting to be cut," or not wanting to sacrifice sexual activity in their prime. They roll the dice, hoping that once their cancers are in remission, recurrence will never surface.

Those who select or undergo radiation have a few pluses going for them. Unlike surgery patients, they can avoid the anxieties some associate with anesthesia. And their procedures can usually be done on an outpatient basis. Under normal circumstances, they can continue pursuing their usual activities following treatment, something busy people find appealing. But it should be noted that radiation can be fatiguing, and many men commonly choose to reduce their work schedules.

If you are considering radiation, you must be aware of one caveat. You may not be eligible for prostate cancer surgery if in the past you have had any radiation treatment of the prostate. That is because the damaging effects on the tissues from radiation can make a surgical procedure very difficult to perform without possibly causing a significant injury to the rectum, urinary sphincter, or other vital local structures.

Let's take a look at radiation today. Modern radiation can be administered by external beam therapy or seed implantation (also called brachytherapy). Sometimes a combination of the two is called for.

From a historical perspective, suffice it to say that fledgling attempts at radiation dating back to the 1930s and 1940s were crude yet promising. They began with X-rays and the use of cobalt and often did more damage and injury to prostate sufferers than can be imagined. The 1970s saw the introduction of seed implantation, but again the results were poor in eradicating prostate cancer. Then the introduction of the linear accelerator in the late 1950s was radiology's "Wright Flyer." A machine was capable for the first time of producing high-energy radiation. Improvements in radiology delivery systems have continued to this day and are analogous to today's most sophisticated aircraft as compared to the Wright Flyer.

Radiologists use a scale to measure doses of radiation energy. It's called the Gray scale (Gy), named for its inventor, Louis Gray, a British radiologist. Treating prostate cancer requires a minimum of 70 Gy. All you need to know here is that the cancer "cure" (or "control") rate increases as the strength (Gy number) increases. So, new technologies, capable of delivering more than 70 Gy—say, 80 Gy or more—promise better chances of knocking out the cancer cells rapidly and effectively.

In preparing for radiation therapy, doctors may suggest a temporary hormonal treatment course. Recent studies at Harvard have shown that temporary hormone therapy prior to X-ray therapy can produce much better results than radiation therapy alone.

Of vital concern to so many patients is the question of sexual potency. Which procedure, surgery or radiation, offers the best chance for continued potency? Is one riskier than the other? Following surgery—a radical prostatectomy—the patient will immediately lose sexual function. There are no exceptions. But—and this is a good "but"—if the surgeon is able to perform nerve sparing during the operation, sexual potency has a good chance to return! In some cases it may occur quickly, but in most instances it can take up to a year and a half to two years. Even if the patient has difficulty getting an erection, there are many remedies currently available to solve the problem of erectile dysfunction (ED).

The patient receiving radiation does not lose his potency immediately following the procedure. He will likely retain sexual function for the next several years. But within two to three years, patients will likely notice a gradual decline in potency—a steady inability to have erections. Many men have real difficulty in performing sexually by five years' time. Natural ED deteriorates as much as 40 to 50 percent from baseline levels in patients within five years. That is a fact not brought out forthrightly in many communications to patients!

Medications like Viagra can often help in these instances of ED. In fact, Dr. Burnett suggests that products like Viagra can be tried in all instances of ED. Scientists continue to work every day on new procedures to deal with sexual dysfunction. At the same time, they remain optimistic that the future path in urological research is bright and that eventually their discoveries will lead to the development of new therapies and vaccines that will eventually help preserve erectile function in the course of treating prostate cancer.

External Beam Radiation

Commonly asked questions about external beam radiation include the following:

"What will external beam radiation do to my quality of life and my lifestyle? And what are the side effects?"

"What will external beam therapy do to my sex life?"

"What will external beam radiation do to my continence?"

"Can I count on external beam therapy to get rid of my cancer for good?"

External beam radiation (shooting the beam from *outside* the body) is the first effective method of delivering radiation in prostate cancer, using an approach called conventional therapy. The accelerator shoots a high-energy dose of 70 Gy over a period of seven weeks, every weekday, with time off on the weekends to allow the patient to rest and for the body to recover and adjust to the radiation treatment.

The targets include the prostate and seminal vesicles. It's up to the skill of the doctor to protect the tissues in proximity to the targets—specifically, the bladder, the rectum, and the urethra. Because conventional therapy irradiates a kind of square box shape around the targets, the delicate tissues of the bladder, rectum, and urethra become very vulnerable to radiation damage. And therein lies the great dilemma—how to irradiate the cancer cells while at the same time protecting the normal tissues? Thus there can be immediate side effects with external beam radiation, such as bleeding, diarrhea, bowel urgency, and urinary frequency. Delivering high enough Gy to kill the cancer cells with conventional radiation can cause many complications.

But there has been good news in the form of the 3D conformal radiation therapy (3D-CRT). Using computers and CT scans, scientists can produce a more accurate delivery system. The prostate is measured in three dimensions, and radiation can focus "inside the box," come in closer, and reduce the hitting of vulnerable areas. This has greatly reduced the risk of side effects and has allowed an increase in Gy or radiation strength, thus increasing the kill level of cancer cells.

Next is a still more accurate delivery system, intensity-modulated radiation therapy (IMRT). IMRT further delineates the target area using computerized algorithms, allowing radiologists to vary intensities of radiation throughout the target area. This sophisticated approach allows the radiation to come within a single centimeter of the prostate gland while protecting the adjacent tissues. Extraordinary precision means that oncologists can deliver knockout blows to the cancer by being able to strike with high doses of radiation—as much as 81, 86, or even 91 Gy—while keeping serious side effects to a minimum.

IMRT equipment is still expensive and so is not yet available at all major prostate cancer centers. If you choose radiation to treat prostate cancer, the best course is to find out what centers can provide 3D-CRT with IMRT. You may have to travel to a center offering this state-of-the-art option, but consider that you only have one life to live and you may well want to live it free of prostate cancer.

Seed Implantation

Commonly asked questions about seed implantation include the following:

"If I have seeds, how long will I have to be away from my job?"

"How do I know if I am a candidate for seeds?"

"Will seeds interfere with my ability to have sex?"

"Will seeds have any effect on my continence?"

We have already described how radiation can be delivered from *outside* the body, with external beam radiation. Seed implantation delivers radiation from *within* the body.

Doctors also refer to seed implantation as brachytherapy or interstitial therapy. In this treatment, radioactive seeds or pellets are placed inside the prostate gland. The surgeon then bombards the cancer cells with the explosive radiation rays while trying to reduce collateral damage to the surrounding structures.

The implantation of radioactive iodine or palladium seeds is almost always permanent. The tiny seeds are held in minuscule titanium capsules and each seed emits a low dosage of radioactive energy. The effect on cancer cells will depend on total cumulative dosage. Whether the seeds are iodine or palladium, they are time-released over many months. In most cases, patients can go home the same day and are able to resume normal activities.

Sometimes intense brachytherapy treatment is suggested to deal with very large, advanced, or recurring tumors. Here a temporary high dosage rate (HDR) of iridium (a brittle silver metallic element) implant is used. Patients are hospitalized for thirty hours, during which time high-energy radiation is delivered into the prostate. HDR is used in conjunction with external beam therapy under local anesthesia.

If you are considering seed implantation, there is something else to be aware of. The anatomy of your prostate gland is of major importance. Large prostates are difficult to saturate safely with seeds. If yours weighs under forty grams, that is perfect. But if it is heavier than that, you risk acute urinary retention. In some cases, seeds can cause tissue swelling. Consequently, the urethra can be squeezed, preventing you from urinating. To avoid this issue, the oncologist does a precise configuration of the prostate to determine if it is too big for seed implants. If it is, hormone therapy may be tried to help shrink the prostate. One major issue associated with brachytherapy is whether the seed implants emit radiation that could be hazardous to others in the vicinity of the patient. For instance, the irradiated grandfather may be told that he cannot hold his grandchild for some time after this therapy!

In sum, patients diagnosed with localized early-stage cancer will want to weigh the pluses and minuses offered by radiation therapy against those offered by a radical prostatectomy before making the very personal decision of how to deal with their prostate cancer.

11

Elliott Halio

Choice May Not Be in the Cards: Staying Alive Is the Ace Up Your Sleeve!

Elliott Halio graduated from Syracuse University in 1952, served with the U.S. Marine Corps during the Korean conflict, went on to study law at Duke University, and earned his J.D. degree in 1957. Elliott married and settled down in Charleston, South Carolina, where he began building his law practice. Today, he practices with his son, Andrew, in their firm, Halio and Halio. Father and son have now worked together for twenty-six years. Elliott Halio's wife, Frances, taught school and is now retired. At the time of this interview, in February 2008, Elliott was seventy-seven.

He became the first associate municipal judge in Charleston, then in 1963 moved up to become municipal judge. After three and a half years, he left public office to devote more time to his private law practice. He became president of the local bar association, helped establish the Young Lawyers' section of the South Carolina State Bar Association, and in the late 1970s became a member of the South Carolina State Bar Association's executive committee. Today, his firm specializes in defending doctors and hospitals in medical malpractice cases.

Elliott has always been into sports. "These days I play quite a bit of golf. It's a throwback from high school where I played all the sports. Basketball, baseball, football. And when I got to college I played a year at basketball, intramurals, of course. And in the Marine Corps, well it was always run, run, run. But when I got to my senior year at Duke Law, I became very ill. I had a ruptured appendix that put me in the hospital for forty-five days. I wound up with a blood clot in one of my legs.

"Then I came to Charleston and became the patient of a very caring doctor, and with his help I set up a schedule to get physical check-ups at least once a year. That started back in 1959. And it was prompted by the fact that I had been ill and had been diagnosed with Crohn's disease, or ileitis [inflammation of the lower intestine]. I had numerous problems with it; in fact, it led to three abdominal surgeries. So I was very much aware of the need for annual check-ups.

"In the seventies I got lucky and had three excellent doctors here in Charleston looking after me. They were giving me thorough physical exams—the whole works. In the late nineties, my primary physician began giving me PSAs, and the numbers were in the range of 1.2 or 1.3 but no more. Then in 2005, the PSA moved up to 3. Still, my internist told me that was okay. And doctors at the VA hospital confirmed the number. I had been going there, too, because they were keeping tabs on me to make sure I wasn't having any more problems with blood clotting. It was about this time that I found I was starting to have some urination problems at night. The urologist gave me some medication to control that, but the urinary issue persisted. I just knew something was not right.

"In the spring of 2006, I had moved on to a new urologist who was trained at Johns Hopkins, and he discovered that my PSA had jumped to 7! Again, the VA hospital verified the results—it was indeed 7. My urologist told me that a prostate biopsy was needed. I didn't find the actual procedure that bad. But the results were. It proved to be positive in eight out of ten cores! The Gleason, they said, was 6. I wasn't shocked when I got the news that I had prostate cancer. For some reason I didn't get upset or panicky.

I just told myself this was something we're gonna have to take care of. I didn't like it. But there it was. It had to be done."

Elliott's new urologist felt previous doctors should have kept a closer watch over his prostate condition. He felt Elliott's problem should have been caught earlier and that his chances for better outcomes might have been sacrificed as a result. Said Elliott, "The urologist went over the options of radiation and seeds with me, and he talked about surgery. Then he handed me a medical book by Dr. Patrick Walsh of Johns Hopkins on dealing with prostate cancer [*Dr. Patrick Walsh's Guide to Surviving Prostate Cancer*]. He even told me what chapters to focus on. He said concentrate on the ones from radiation, simply because he said that at my age, surgery was probably not the best option for me. So I read about surgery, read about radiation, and the chapter on seeds. One of the reasons why I didn't like the idea of surgery was because over the years I had had ten major operations. I didn't want any more surgery. I just didn't want it. And it was very easy, when I read the book and found that radiation was probably the ideal thing for me, it was an easy decision to make, and I made it."

Elliott did not feel the need to share news of his cancer with anyone other than family members. "That's right. I didn't tell anybody else. And then I found out that my wife had told her sister. I got very upset about that because I didn't think it was anybody else's business except mine. Later on, I realized that it was kind of a narrow attitude to take and not to be concerned about it. Aside from reading the Walsh book I didn't see the need to do further research. I didn't go online. My son, Andy, doesn't show emotions particularly, but I know he was concerned. I know him well enough to know that. But outwardly he didn't say or do anything. My daughter was very upset and said so. She was very outspoken about it. She was very worried about me."

Elliott Halio describes his experience undergoing radiation treatments. "My urologist introduced me to my radiation oncologist. She turned out to be a peach. She is not only an excellent physician but a caring one, too. She sat down with me and spent a full *hour* explaining what radiation was all about. She was very interested in hearing how I felt about radiation and my concerns. She went into the treatments very thoroughly—forty-four treatments, one per day for five days a week. What side effects might occur due to the radiation. And I was prepared. I was prepared ahead of time.

"First of all, before radiation began, there was hormone treatment to deal with. I got a shot. I don't remember the name of it, but, as the doctors put it, it was supposed to put the cancer cells to sleep, so they'd become easy targets for the radiation and so they wouldn't multiply. I had that shot in November 2006. I had the second shot in April 2007. All in all, hormone treatments totally took eight months. That's when I started having hot flashes. I lost all the hair on my chest. Every bit of it, and whether the rash that I subsequently developed on my thighs was due to the hormones or the treatment that followed, I don't know. I also remember becoming very hungry. I mean, I ate anything and everything in sight, putting on a quick ten pounds which I have yet to success-fully shed. But those hot flashes—that was not a pleasant experience. And it made me think of what my wife went through and how I belittled it. Well, I can sympathize with women now. Because when I went through it—boy, are they uncomfortable. And you never know when those damned flashes are gonna hit you! You're sitting there just as nice as can be and all of a sudden . . . *wham*! You are sweating away. You can't wait for this thing to be over. My wife was somewhat sympathetic, but then the two of us would just sit there and laugh. We didn't worry about it. Maybe Frances was getting even."

Elliott explains that the preparation for his radiation was precise and the plan allowed for an uninterrupted workday fol-lowing his daily treatment. "They laid out a treatment schedule for me, which I had to approve. The radiologist technician took measurements needed to place me correctly on the table, then drew some very dark 'X' markings at various places on the table. [The idea is to allow for precise alignment to direct the radiation beams as the patient undergoes treatment.] Importantly, the doc-tors made certain that all of this fit into my schedule so I could keep my practice going without interruption. I decided the best thing for me was to take treatments early in the morning. They started at seven-fifteen. Positioning [under the machine] took about ten minutes. The radiation treatment itself would only last ten minutes, so twenty minutes in all. The urologist put three seeds into my prostate gland so that the technicians could direct the radiation [beams] directly where they needed to go. So I'd get to the hospital at seven, start the treatment at seven-fifteen, and I'd be out of there and at my office by eight at the latest."

When he went to work, Elliott says he felt fine. His energy level was up, but as the day wore on fatigue began setting in. "It really hit me soon as I got home. I felt myself getting drained, and early in the evenings I would just go out like a light. Toward the end of the radiation regimen I have to say I felt weak as a kitten. I also found that radiation was causing me to urinate often. At night, I had to go frequently. But I had to find a way in the daytime so it wouldn't interfere with my work. That could be a problem in the kind of work I do. You don't try a case for one or two days. You try a case over one or two weeks sometimes. So you have to be resourceful here. So I had to go to the judges in private and tell them I had a lot of urgency and I never knew exactly when it was gonna be, but when it came, I had to leave the courtroom *immediately*. The radiation was causing me to go often. And there were two judges because there were two different trials, and the judges said, 'Just raise your hand and give us the signal, and we'll take a little recess, and you can go to the bathroom.' So that's what I did. I would raise my hand and take a pee break. The judges would smile. They were very understanding and good about that.

"My work is what kept me from even thinking about the cancer. Once I left the hospital after having that radiation, I got to my office and started focusing on my work. I never thought about cancer. I never thought about the radiation. In fact, I was making appointments at seven-thirty, eight o'clock in the morning, not realizing that I couldn't be there because I had to be at the hospital. Today, I'm feeling fine. I have a medication that I take to prevent me from having any urinary problems at night. Truth is, most of the time I don't wake up in the middle of the night to go. If I do, I maybe go, it's one time at the most."

What would Elliott like to pass on to prostate cancer patients and their families? "You've got to accept the fact that you have to do something about the problem. Once you make a choice of how you want the problem treated, and once you embark on the treatment, it's easy after that. Accept the problem, don't turn your back on it, don't deny you've got it. Just go in and do whatever it is to stay alive. And do what I learned to do—keep busy! If you're among the less fortunate ones who have a short time to live, you'd better enjoy every minute you have and do the things you've always wanted to do. Just do it and live!"

The Doctor's Notebook

Elliott Halio's account typifies that of a patient undergoing external beam radiation therapy for prostate cancer. I am impressed by his fortitude and optimism amid the effects of this treatment on his bodily functions. His decision to pursue radiation therapy was understandable, and having undergone so many surgeries in the past along with his slightly older age of diagnosis were grounds to proceed in this fashion. A younger man with likely far less risks to undergo an additional surgery perhaps would have been better suited to pursue the radical prostatectomy option. Elliott's case history makes the point that no one intervention is right for everyone. There are multiple treatment options for early-stage prostate cancer, and decisions need to be tailored based on the extent of disease, patient health status and expectations of longevity, and patient preferences. Thus every alternative is right in the right circumstances. Most important of all is the right decision to move forward in discussions with competent and caring consultants to be informed and get treated.

Prescriptive Information

Expectant Management
In the past, doctors used the term "wait and see" when a decision is reached to withhold treatment altogether unless the cancer becomes more aggressive. In today's medical parlance, the term

has been upgraded to "expectant management," reflecting a more proactive course in following the disease. The procedure calls for an active course of surveillance of the patient's condition and for periodic check-ups that can include DREs, PSAs, and, if needed, biopsy. In recent times, doctors have found that in many men diagnosed with cancers, the cancers are small enough to pose no imminent threat to their lives. In those cases, the risks associated with treatment and possible loss of a comfortable lifestyle may make less sense than proceeding with immediate intervention, and so a patient may elect a course of expectant management. Such a course is also a viable choice for older men who are too ill or who don't want to undergo the rigors of treatment.

PART III

Warnings and Conflicts

12

Yohannes Abate

Sidestepping a Rush to Judgment

At the time of this interview in 2007, Yohannes Abate, at sixty-seven, was a geographer working for the Department of Defense. He first came to the United States in 1970 from his native Ethiopia as a graduate student at the University of Maryland. His story spotlights the current controversy on whether widespread testing leads to overdiagnosis and unnecessary risk for men with minimal prostate cancer.

Yohannes says that since his U.S. Army days he's always tried staying in good physical shape and got annual medical check-ups starting at age thirty-eight. He admits to knowing little about the prostate until the early 1990s when his primary doctor began offering him DREs and PSA tests. His numbers stayed steady, less than 2, until 2003, when they began slowly climbing. They moved from less than 2 to 2.1, then to 2.3 by 2005. He got concerned because he found himself running frequently to the bathroom. That's when he began tracking his PSAs on a graph.

In October 2006, while accompanying his wife for her physical exam at George Washington University (GW), Yohannes noticed a sign offering free prostate testing. When he underwent the test, he discovered his PSA remained at 2.3. But in April 2007, when he returned to GW for his annual physical, the number had jumped to 3.1. His doctor grew concerned because in the short period of time between November and April the PSA had moved up rapidly. Still, his primary doctor told him not to be alarmed because his number remained below 4—considered within the normal range. But nonetheless she wanted him to be seen by a urologist for a biopsy to be sure.

That very day Yohannes was sitting in the urologist's office, prepared for the worst.

"The doctor began by telling me that of fourteen [core] samples taken, two had shown positive. But he went on to say I shouldn't worry because over the next five years they might never grow. We also talked about options. Seeds, radiation, various other possible therapies. My own research on prostate cancer did not encourage me to consider radiation or these other options. I became convinced from what I read that if you catch prostate cancer early as possible, as long as the cancer was contained in the prostate, the best solution was to get it out. Of course, I did worry about the outcomes of surgery, but I also felt that your life was more important than whether you would have incontinence or impotence.

"The urologist was a surgeon and said he could do laparoscopic surgery on me at GW. He told me he did two or three a week and so far he'd done them for several months. But when I realized he was only at GW less than a year, I didn't feel confident even though he told me he was getting pretty good at it. I decided not to talk it over with my wife because she herself had been diagnosed with breast cancer, so I didn't want to add my problems to hers."

Yohannes had not made up his mind to proceed with the operation. He kept pondering, wondering if he would be making the right move. "This was the very early stage of my decision, whether to do the surgery or not. I went back to the urologist and asked him to do a risk factor analysis, and he did. After he consulted nomograms [a mathematical tool, similar to the Partin tables], he told that my chance of recovery was ninety-four percent.

That was a pretty good number, and we scheduled the surgery for the middle of August 2007."

Yohannes still felt uncomfortable and continued his research. "I was reading over the Scardino book [*Dr. Peter Scardino's Prostate Book*], and in it the authors kept pounding away at getting a second opinion. And if you decide to do laparoscopic surgery, you'd better get the best doctor—absolutely the best! And so I decided to find a doctor to give me that second opinion."

Yohannes wound up at Johns Hopkins, where he was scheduled for an appointment with Dr. Burnett. "I checked the Internet and read about Dr. Burnett. I told myself he is at one of the leading institutes of urology in the world. And so an opinion from one of their doctors was what I really needed.

"Dr. Burnett looked at the write-up on the biopsy and said this cancer was really at the very, very early stage and that I should take my time and not worry a lot, but he wanted to see the slides. And when he got them he said the Hopkins pathology findings were identical to the GW findings. The good thing was that GW was up to snuff. Dr. Burnett said emphatically again there was nothing to worry about. He did not say yes or no. I like that. He was leaving it to me. Letting me make an informed decision, and I liked that. I had enough information to go along with his diagnosis. Dr. Burnett alleviated my anxieties. Absolutely. He said my cancer is minimal as it can get, and I shouldn't worry about it. It's as minimal as it could get. I could watch this, and he could help me watch this situation. And so on my way back from Johns Hopkins I had a great sense of relief. Within a couple of days of the meeting with Dr. Burnett, I called my doctor at GW and said cancel the surgery!

"Now that I've been through this, I would tell other people you must get a second opinion. The second opinion is the best decision I think I ever made. Absolutely, the best decision I have ever made!"

Update as of September 2009: Yohannes Abate is retired. He has never had surgery and continues with expectant management. He says his PSA has not risen further, and he is feeling fine, enjoying excellent health, and thriving in his retirement.

The Doctor's Notebook

Yohannes Abate's prostate cancer story typifies a fairly common-place management dilemma today. In the course of his prostate health check-ups, a prostate cancer diagnosis was made, although its significance was in question. But his good diligence was rewarded only with a diagnosis that seemed to present an ambiguous situation. His PSA velocity, or rate of change of PSA values over time, which is a valuable diagnostic tool to facilitate early prostate cancer diagnoses, understandably prompted his biopsy. But the ensuing diagnosis was perplexing. Was he diagnosed early with a major prostate cancer presentation, or was he just found to have clinically low-profile prostate cancer amid a proactive good health program? The dilemma is the finding of prostate cancer that rates as a low amount or aggressiveness level, which could suggest a cancer that may never spread in his lifetime. It is true that many men will die *with* prostate cancer and not *from* it. After thoroughly understanding the minimal extent of his prostate cancer diagnosis and the possibility that it would not necessarily be a threat to his life, Yohannes made an informed decision to proceed with an expectant management protocol.

This story strikes me as one of how to gain emotional fortitude and perspective. Yohannes's emotional distress came about not only because of his prostate cancer diagnosis but also because his wife was grappling with a cancer diagnosis at the same time. He says today that he regrets not having sought emotional support from those around him—only his doctors—while he pursued a logical process of thorough information gathering. It might have eased his anxiety. Yohannes describes the process he was carrying out as tantamount to "getting a second opinion," although the additional opinion may well be considered his own. I credit this man for learning as much as possible about his prostate cancer diagnosis and his treatment options in order to make that informed decision—and, of course, for coming by to see me for a true and formal second medical opinion.

Prescriptive Information

Causes and Risk Factors of Prostate Cancer

To understand what causes prostate cancer, let's first define the term. Put simply, cancer is a malignant tumor or growth that occurs when normal cells mutate into "bad" cells and multiply uncontrollably to the point where they overwhelm and destroy healthy cells. Why does this happen and under what circumstances?

The answer is contained in three letters that you are undoubtedly familiar with: DNA. It is our genetic "blueprint," the vital information contained in the nucleus of every cell. DNA carries all our hereditary information. Think of it this way. DNA tells each of our cells to make specific building blocks. These blocks then stretch out as strings of chemicals, and scientists attach letters to each block to identify them. Change one letter or block and you can change the whole arrangement. A gene is a particular sequence of DNA codes that orchestrates how a single protein (the complex essential structure of each of our cells) is built. This genetic code is the body's greatest asset, and the body tries to defend it like the Alamo. Every time a cell divides the genetic code must be replicated *perfectly*. There is an army of "fact checkers" (mismatch-repair genes and tumor-suppressor genes) to correct any deficiencies. Most of the time, these "fact checkers" are up to the task. But there are instances when they can be defeated, allowing the DNA to become damaged. *And all cancers are caused by damage to the DNA.*

What causes DNA damage? One instance is when a tiny damage to a single cell is "missed" by the "fact checkers," and that cell may remain hidden deep within the body for years or even decades. Over time, the cell mutates; others follow suit, creating an environment in which these cancerous cells grow to such an army that they crush the body's normal defenses. In other instances, the "fix-it" genes are unable to fend off threats from outside the body—environmental causes. For instance, ultraviolet light can lead to skin cancer. Chemical compounds in cigarette smoke—even secondary smoke—can cause lung cancer. In sum, whenever DNA in our cells is subjected to attack from within or without the body, mutations of the cells take place, leading to the development of cancer.

What then are the risk factors for prostate cancer that we must be aware of? Three of the greatest are age, race, and family history.

Age: The incidence of prostate cancer rises dramatically with age. The reason is that cell mutations occur gradually and over time, as oxidative damage takes place. For American men forty to fifty-nine, the risk of developing prostate cancer is 1 in 50. For men age sixty to seventy-nine, the risk factor is 1 in 7. And when a man reaches his mid- to late seventies, the risk that he will develop prostate cancer is seven times more than a man in his forties. That works out to his risk being *130 times* more than a man in his mid- to late fifties. Over a lifetime, an American man's risk of developing prostate cancer is estimated to be 1 in 6.

Race: African American men have the highest risk of prostate cancer of any ethnic group in the world. The number of black men per hundred thousand who develop the disease is 40 percent higher than the number of white Americans. And those who do develop prostate cancer are likely to have more severe cases and are more likely to die from it. Not only that, but even after African American men have been treated, they frequently have a recurrence of the disease. Researchers continue to probe for the reasons why. But preliminary investigations suggest that the causes relate to genetic susceptibility, diet, and inadequate exposure to vitamin D, a protector against cancer.

The dire prostate cancer statistics for African Americans would be even worse but for the fact that they are also at higher risk for other critical health issues: hypertension and coronary artery disease. In other words, black men generally do not live long enough to make it to old age, so their lifetime risk of prostate cancer is about 13 percent compared to 16 percent for white Americans. The sad truth is that their lifetime risk of developing prostate cancer is lower because they are likely to die of some other illness before they live long enough to suffer from prostate cancer.

Hispanic and Asian Americans are less likely to develop prostate cancer than white American men.

Family history: If your father or brother has had prostate cancer, your risk of developing the disease is 2 to 2½ times greater than the general population's. That means that instead of your chances of developing cancer being 1 in 6, they double to 1 in 3. Suppose three of your family members developed the disease (for example, your father and two brothers); if so, you are in the category of having "hereditary prostate cancer." That would be true, too, if prostate cancer occurred in three generations in your family (say, your grandfather, father, a cousin, or a brother). Or if two of your relatives developed prostate cancer at an early age (younger than fifty-five), you can tell the doctor you have a history of prostate cancer in your family. In any of these cases, the risk that you will develop the disease can be as high as 50 percent.

Straight Talk and Myth Busting

A lot of guys who don't have their facts straight will buy into assumptions and tall tales. Unfortunately, it can really cost them. Here are some that frequently make the rounds:

Myth: An elevated PSA always means you have prostate cancer. A "normal" PSA means you don't.

Truth: PSA levels can be affected by things other than prostate cancer. For example, PSA can rise because of prostatitis or BPH (benign prostatic hyperplasia, or prostate enlargement). You can have prostate cancer and low PSA levels. Nevertheless, so far the PSA test is the best tool we have to find prostate cancer early.

Myth: Even if your PSA level is high, a negative (no cancer indicator) prostate biopsy means you definitely do not have cancer.

Truth: Wrong! Though doctors try to get as many representative samples of the prostate during biopsy, small tumors can be hard to find. The doctor may recommend another biopsy.

Myth: Removal of the prostate or treatment with radiation will guarantee a cure for prostate cancer.

Truth: Wrong! There are no lifetime guarantees. Retreatment may be needed in some difficult cases.

Myth: BPH is inevitable for most men. When the prostate becomes cancerous, cutting it out will remove the problem.

Truth: BPH does not mean the prostate is cancerous. The enlarged prostate is treatable and need not result in prostate cancer.

Myth: Sex is not good for the prostate.

Truth: The prostate is perfectly happy if you have a regular, loving sex life. Recent epidemiological studies at Johns Hopkins suggest that increased sexual activity offers protection against the occurrence of prostate cancer. The thought is that men who have frequent ejaculations may alter the composition of prostatic fluid and actually lower the concentration of potentially harmful chemicals that have been linked to prostate cancer. In short, increased sexual activity may offer protection against the disease. In fact, celibate men have the highest incidence of prostate cancer.

Myth: Prostate cancer means you will be permanently disabled, unable to work again.

Truth: Many men continue to work during treatment. If you undergo a prostatectomy you may have to take four to six weeks off to recover from surgery, but you should be able to resume your normal activity afterward.

Myth: Impotence always follows all treatment.

Truth: That is not true for all treatments! After a prostatectomy, potency may be lost for a time. If the nerve bundles are spared, some men regain potency quickly, while for others it may take time while the nerves recover. But in any event, there are generally options that enable patients to resume sexual activity within a short time.

Myth: Prostatitis can cause prostate cancer.

Truth: Wrong! Prostatitis is a common cause of urinary tract infection in men. An estimated 25 percent of all men who see a doctor for urological problems have symptoms of prostatitis. Most of these conditions are treatable with antibiotics. But prostatitis is not a precursor of prostate cancer.

13

Earl G. Graves Sr.

Stern Advice to Young African American Men: Listen Up!

Fortune magazine has named Earl G. Graves Sr. one of the most powerful and influential African Americans in corporate America. He is the founder and publisher of *Black Enterprise*, one of the country's leading magazines devoted to African American business professionals, entrepreneurs, and policymakers in both the public and private sectors. He is a vigilant forger of equal opportunity for black men and women in the nation. When we spoke to Earl Graves in 2006, he was seventy-one and at the top of his game.

Earl grew up in the Bedford-Stuyvesant section of Brooklyn, New York, and says he is ever grateful for having two incredible parents who modeled strong values and held high expectations for him from the day he was born. He graduated with a B.A. in economics from Morgan State University and at twenty-five became an administrative assistant to Senator Robert F. Kennedy. There his focus on economic development and health care, particularly as it related to black Americans, left an indelible mark on his life. He is a proud man wedded to the mission of uplifting his people economically and in matters of health. Today, Earl Graves and his wife, Barbara, live in Westchester, New York, and have three sons and eight grandchildren.

Earl credits the success of *Black Enterprise* to his wife of fifty years and to his sons, all of whom are partners in the business. In 2006, Earl G. Graves Jr., the oldest, became president and CEO, while Earl Sr. retains the title of chairman and publisher. Earl Sr.'s vigor and energy belie his age. He remains a hard-driving executive who enjoys handsome shirts and splashy ties. His considerable height, muttonchops, and large-rimmed glasses make him hard to miss. The offices of *Black Enterprise* on New York's Fifth Avenue are trendy and luxurious, with a carpeted spiral staircase between floors providing an option to the elevators. Accolades cover the walls and trophies abound in celebration of Earl Sr.'s achievements, attesting to his highly visible statement that he is indeed "the man."

Earl Sr.'s prowess in business and education has sent him into orbit in a world peopled with corporate executives, political and civic leaders, wealthy entertainers, sports legends, and college presidents. He served as CEO of Pepsi-Cola of Washington, D.C., the largest minority-controlled Pepsi franchise in the United States. He has sat on boards including AMR (American Airlines), Aetna, and Howard University. He is a trustee of Tuskegee University, has received honorary degrees from fifty-three colleges and universities, and his alma mater, Morgan State, renamed its business school the Earl G. Graves School of Business and Management.

Earl Sr. will tell you that working for Robert Kennedy awakened him to the need for health care. "Growing up, we didn't have the money for preventive health care. It wasn't even in our vocabulary. And then my father died of a heart attack at the age of forty-eight! That's when I came to understand that when you reach forty or thereabouts, you'd better start checking on your health. As I developed relationships with faculty members and administrators at a number of predominately African American schools, and even became a trustee of a few, like Howard, I met a lot of doctors and started learning more and more about health issues and the inequities that exist in health care—especially as it relates to African Americans. Given my father's early death, I stayed focused on making sure my own health was in good shape."

That so many African American men get prostate cancer first made an impact on Earl Sr. when he went to a Morgan State University homecoming, where five of his good friends told him they had the disease. He thought he was the only one in the group who didn't. But he was wrong. Shortly thereafter, Earl Sr. learned that he too had prostate cancer!

What struck him was the stunning realization that prostate cancer is an equal-opportunity disease. It shows no respect for who you are. Prominent men are just as likely to be struck down as ordinary ones. "I was shocked. The word 'cancer' just gives you a punch in the stomach. I told my doctors, 'Do whatever it is you have to do.' I was very positive that they would work it out. Of course, it helped that they were very encouraging. It felt great to be told that the chances of survival are ninety-nine percent if you are diagnosed early enough. Thank goodness, in my case, it was early.

"Going back twenty-five years, I started getting exams for the prostate and having colonoscopies on a regular basis. I was in my forties when I suddenly discovered I had a high PSA on three or four occasions. It would go down and spike again. So the doctor thought it was either an infection that I was going to have on occasion or it was cancer! Years later the actual exam that showed I had cancer cells in my prostate was the result of a routine check-up. The men who made the determination were Dr. Aaron Jackson, who was head of urology at Howard University, and Dr. LaSalle Leffall, the chief of surgery. Both of them urged me to validate their findings by going over to Johns Hopkins and having Dr. Burnett take a look. He is one of the leading doctors in this field and in this country. I was a trustee at Howard and there was a deference paid me, which I must say was comforting in its own right because everybody kept saying, 'We're going to work your way through this thing.' I went over and had a meeting with Dr. Burnett. He evaluated my situation, did the test and the biopsy samples came back and they were indeed cancerous."

Earl Sr. says he had complete faith in all three of his physicians. "All these doctors thought that surgery was the way to go. And so in March 2004 I had Dr. Burnett remove my prostate. I'm not sure what the success rate is, but I've been cancer-free ever since.

And of course I show up for the PSA every three months now, and I always have an annual physical.

"The outcomes following the prostatectomy were splendid. I regard them as a blessing. I was so very fortunate that the issue of incontinence worked out for me. I always had a weak bladder to begin with. So I began wearing pads for a period of time, but guess what? That problem has diminished! Medication helped. It takes time to resolve incontinence and potency issues. You have to give the body the needed chance to heal."

Although it turned out well, Earl Sr. remembers the uncertainty of that time and how key his wife, Barbara, was in seeing him through it. "I've said it publicly, and I've said it to her privately: the best thing that ever happened to me is my wife. That was true before I had cancer, but it was never more true than when I was going through this. I called her my own private Florence Nightingale. She was very optimistic. She didn't collapse. I know some people close to the patient can become more upset and depressed than the patient himself. That was not true of my wife. She remained completely supportive, and I kept her involved. From the beginning, she knew about every test, every result, every option and the risks attached to them, including the chances of my having impotency or incontinence after surgery. So we both dealt with all of that together and having her by my side every step of the way made all the difference in the world for me."

Earl Sr.'s perspective is that black men's lack of participation in the health-care system has deep roots. "Many ask why so many African American men avoid early screening for prostate cancer when the disease has reached epidemic proportions. The answer is complicated.

"First of all, the whole environment around prostate cancer messes with our egos and our ideas of manhood. We have to get past our hang-ups about possible aftereffects of the disease. As men, we kid around, but we want to think of ourselves as virile. We want to think of ourselves as being able to rip and roar at age seventy, which is unrealistic. Second, I am part of the first generation of black men able to afford consistent health care, which historically we were denied in this country. And the access to health care predated the access to the capital that would pay for it, so we're still in the process of breaking generations of poor health habits that grew out of a lack of options.

"Black neighborhoods across this country are still fighting for healthier local food choices, health education in schools, and better local health services for preventive care. There are some in the black community who still don't trust our health-care system because of incidents like the Tuskegee Syphilis Experiment. For forty years, the U.S. government duped four hundred black men into believing they were being treated for 'bad blood' and experimented on them, knowing they had syphilis and they would die. That just ended in 1972! So black men's resistance to health care is very complicated.

"But I really think the root of it with prostate cancer is the manhood issue. Men attach their sense of manhood to virility, and our society has challenged the manhood of black men in so many different ways for so many years that these men are not going to be eager to do anything that they see as a threat to their manhood. Some see the treatment of prostate cancer as just that. I think the key is to get them to understand that being a real man has more to do with how you conduct yourself than anything else. I do think things are improving. There's mentoring going on in black churches, in schools, community centers, even through magazines like mine to openly speak to the issue. But the problem is the word is not getting out there fast enough, and that's why it's so important for highly visible people to help in the effort.

"It's tough, but it's doable. One of the things I've set as a goal for myself is to reach out to all those million three hundred thousand young African American men sitting in jails—and those who could end up there if somebody doesn't show them another road. We need to let them know they haven't been forgotten, that their lives matter, and that we still need them in the black community and in the world. We need them to get their lives together—to get educated, to set legitimate goals, get jobs and work hard, support their children and model better lives for them, a better model than they may have had for themselves. It comes back to this notion of manhood—what it is and what it isn't—and good health is the foundation for all of that."

Earl Graves Sr. has issued a clarion call for all black men over the age of forty (and even younger if there's a family history of the disease) to have an annual rectal exam and a PSA test so that any problem can be detected as early as possible. "It is not about your manhood," says Earl Sr., "it is about your life!"

The Doctor's Notebook

I am overjoyed that Earl Graves Sr. has made a contribution to this book. His disclosure of his health condition and perspectives on health in general carry significant weight, particularly for the African American community.

On one level, he relates his experience as a patient confronting a prostate cancer diagnosis. He shares that the prostate cancer diagnosis was a setback, much as others have acknowledged. Once he was diagnosed with prostate cancer, he accepted it and moved forward with a treatment plan in a most informed way. As he acknowledges further, keys to his success included supportive friends and family, and above all, his wife.

I have identified my interaction with Earl Sr. to be special in many ways. On a basic level, he is my patient. This means that I have the utmost commitment to him with regard to achieving his very best health outcomes. Further, I see in him much of myself, a fellow African American who has encountered various life struggles on the basis of race but who remains very positive about advancing one's self-worth irrespective of this concern. He represents for me a symbol that artificial boundaries can be tested and removed and excellence can be achieved for anybody. Ours is a bond, I think, of mutual admiration and praise.

Earl Sr.'s story offers many messages. That he is African American provides an opportunity to discuss the significance of prostate cancer affecting African Americans. It is recognized that the disease disproportionately affects African Americans. Various explanations have been brought forward to address this issue. Several barriers, ranging from socioeconomic to cultural, are certainly relevant. At the same time, scientific work suggests that there may be a different biological basis for the disease in African Americans. This commitment to learn more about the causes and impact of prostate cancer in the African American community must continue.

I will take this opportunity to offer a few additional thoughts about Earl Sr. as a model individual. I appreciate his focus and commitment on multiple levels to advance not just the health but also the pride of African Americans. Again, it is symbolic that he does what he says and thus his actions speak a thousand words. He is a champion for screening and treatment of prostate cancer particularly among African Americans. Because of his visibility and breadth of interactions in worlds from business to medicine, his ability to champion the cause will continue to be extraordinary. He stresses many messages, perhaps foremost among them an emphasis on the value of education and the inner strength of being properly informed.

Prescriptive Information

The African American Enigma

Every hour in the United States three African American men are told they have prostate cancer. In the next hundred minutes from the time you read this, another African American man will die of the disease. Black men in this country have the highest rate of prostate cancer in the entire world! They are one and a half times more likely to develop the disease and two to three times more likely to die of it than their white counterparts. The statistics are staggering. Why? How can that be?

So far, the answers have eluded frustrated researchers, but they are finally beginning to make inroads. Progress has been slow because, for many complex reasons, African American men have not come forward in sufficient numbers to participate in the very studies aimed at solving the puzzle that can save their lives.

A number of preliminary findings are worthy of note. At the University of Mississippi School of Medicine in Jackson, researchers found that African American men have a higher incidence of a precancerous condition known as high-grade intraepithelial neoplasia (HGPIN) than white males. Because black men are more prone to getting prostate cancer, these researchers believe this higher occurrence of HGPIN may signal changes in the prostate gland becoming cancerous. They also say that even among men with normal PSA levels, men who show high HGPIN levels also have higher PSA measurements. The lead investigator, Dr. Jackson Fowler Jr., says, "The prevalence of cancer and HGPIN [in African American men] is higher and their PSAs tend to be higher."

A study by University of Michigan Health System scientists discovered a gene (MSR1) that plays a significant role in prostate cancer in black Americans. This finding adds to the expanding body of evidence linking the gene mutations as risk factors for the disease. A common frustration among prostate cancer researchers is that samplings in their studies are not sufficiently large because of the reluctance of African Americans to participate.

What we know for certain is that there is a strong hereditary link in prostate cancer. Besides race and ethnicity, men with a father, brother, or son who has had prostate cancer are at greater risk of acquiring the disease. But it's been difficult to nail down the precise genes involved in the cancer until now. Once that is firmly determined, genetic markers should be able to predict with some accuracy just which men are at high risk.

The popular understanding is that the incidence of prostate cancer among blacks in the United States far surpasses the incidence among blacks living in African nations. Accordingly, theories abound to explain the whys. High-fat diets, impoverishment, and at-risk lifestyles are among the common hypotheses. But our view is that caution is advised. Investigations in African nations have been focused primarily on AIDS. Few longitudinal studies have so far been carried out to determine the true occurrence of prostate cancer in African countries. In addition, the number of AIDS-related deaths among a wide range of demographics is so high that it subverts attempts to track those deaths attributable to prostate cancer alone. And so we believe that, as far as the accurate extent of prostate cancer among black men living in Africa is concerned, the jury is still out.

There is a stark irony in the reluctance of so many African American men to participate in research studies aimed at saving them from prostate cancer in light of the fact that the disease among them is epidemic and they could be the prime benefactors. Clearly, the roots of this reluctance lie buried deep within the history of the African American experience in this country, starting from the days of slavery to the fight for civil rights to the notorious Tuskegee study, a forty-year experiment conducted by the U.S. Public Health Service to determine the effects of syphilis on black men who were deprived of treatment and allowed to die. These incidents led to urban legends about hospitals reaching out into black neighborhoods to snatch children for "experiments."

Add to this the African American sensitivity on the issue of manliness and fear of its loss and small wonder the seeds of distrust of the government and of medical institutions bear the fruits of resistance to ethical and legitimate studies that may save African American lives.

The American Cancer Society and the American Urological Association are among those urging black men to be proactive in avoiding the delayed discovery and associated adversities of prostate cancer by undergoing annual screening between the ages of forty and forty-five. That screening includes two tests: a DRE and a PSA test. It urges men to put aside the reluctance and disregard the stigma that may be associated with these examinations.

14

Pat Robertson

Action and Prayer Define His Courage

In mid-February 2003, the familiar face of the host of the Christian Broadcasting Network's popular *700 Club* telecast, Pat Robertson, was missing from the screen. An estimated 63 million subscribers in the United States and millions more in approximately 180 countries around the world learned that Pat Robertson had prostate cancer and had elected to have surgery to rid himself of the scourge and save his life. The news came as a shock to his devoted following and word came to him that countless of them were offering up prayers for his speedy recovery. It was news, he says, that helped sustain him.

Pat Robertson is a global businessman with media holdings in the United States, Asia, the United Kingdom, and Africa. Here in the United States, he is the founder and chairman of the Christian Broadcasting Network (CBN) along with several other broadcasting entities. He established International Family Entertainment, Inc., which was eventually acquired by Disney in 2001 (it is now called ABC Family). He also created the American Center for Law and Justice, a public interest law firm that focuses on pro-life cases nationwide. He is responsible for setting up Operation Blessing International Relief and Development Corporation, a group committed to helping urban populations around the world.

In 1978, Robertson founded Regent University on the site of his CBN headquarters in Virginia Beach. The school offers both undergraduate and graduate degrees as well as a law school. Robertson serves as the chancellor of the university.

Pat Robertson majored in history at Washington and Lee University and graduated magna cum laude with a bachelor of arts degree. He became the university's first person to be commissioned as a Marine second lieutenant. In 1951, during the Korean conflict, he served with the Marines in Japan and Korea. Pat earned a law degree from Yale in 1955 but decided against practicing. Instead, he underwent a religious conversion and attended the New York Theological Seminary, earning a master of divinity degree in 1959. He was ordained a minister of the Southern Baptist Convention in 1961. Soon he was to discover his calling as a religious broadcaster.

In September 1986, Robertson declared his intention to seek the Republican nomination for president of the United States, running on a conservative platform against incumbent vice president George H. W. Bush. His campaign got off to a strong second-place finish in the Iowa caucus, ahead of Bush, but he was unable to remain competitive in his bid once the multiple state primaries were in full swing. His campaign ended before the primaries were concluded. Bush wound up securing the nomination, and Pat Robertson returned to CBN and stayed on as a religious broadcaster and host of the *700 Club*.

Pat Robertson was seventy-eight when we visited with him at CBN headquarters on the Regent University campus. The entrance to the regal colonial-style administration building is splendid, with imposing columns and grand staircases. Much of the credit for the furnishings throughout go to Pat's wife, Adelia "Dede" Elmer. She serves on the board of trustees at Regent and is a long-standing member of the board of directors of CBN. Dede met her husband when she was working on her master's degree in nursing at Yale. The Robertsons have been married for fifty-four years and have four grown children—two sons and two daughters—and fourteen grandchildren.

Pat's office is spacious, resplendent with furnishings that spell pure southern comfort. He is a gracious man with a charismatic smile, and since we were both Marines and prostate cancer survivors, it was an immediate "high five" moment. Pat told me he has always been physically active. "I lift weights and play golf. I used to love to walk, especially in the mountains. I like to ride horses. I've ridden western saddle, English saddle, but primarily English. You know, if you ride jumpers and ride and train dressage horses and are having athletic performances, I can tell you that you're involved, especially with your legs and thighs and core. I'm not in as good a shape as I'd like to be, but I will say I'm passably good."

Pat began taking annual physicals when he turned sixty. "Before that, I didn't have physicals very often. I had a good friend as my family doctor and I would see him from time to time. For me it was strictly a function of insurance policies. They have some pretty large insurance policies for me here and the insurance company wanted me to take physicals. If the insurance company signed you up for multimillion dollars, they want to make sure you're not gonna drop dead. So they have these physicals they ask you to take. I think they started taking those PSAs in the nineties. Just bragging rights I wanted to show how low on the various indices I was and at the same time how macho I was. I considered myself in very good shape. But my doctor didn't particularly want to do a PSA because he said the insurance didn't cover it. He said, 'I don't think you want to afford it.' Finally, I *insisted* he do a PSA. Well, lo and behold . . . it came back with about a 4.4 number! It was enough to set off some alarm bells. My older brother [A. Willis "Tad" Robertson, a stockbroker in Atlanta] died of prostate cancer. And I was there by his bedside when he died. The cancer had spread to his lungs and it spread to his brain! He had radiation. And they thought that they would catch it. But the radiation didn't work! It was just an unfortunate thing that he died . . . and I was there. He was at the time about seventy-seven. So he wasn't exactly a youngster. At the same time, he wasn't in bad physical condition. But this prostate cancer was just more than he could handle. In any event, I *insisted* on this last physical that I had with my doctor . . . I *insisted*. I had taken a blood test and running it through as a PSA. He didn't want to do it, but I insisted that he do it.

"There was no question that prostate cancer runs in our family. You know, if you've had a father or a brother or an uncle who's had it, better get yourself checked out regularly. I have two sons and fourteen grandchildren, and I have encouraged all of them to one day have PSAs. I had no symptoms whatsoever. I was lifting heavy weights in those days. We're talking about leg pressing. I hit two thousand pounds on a leg press and I could do twenty or thirty reps of a thousand pounds, and I had absolutely no symptoms—none! That's often so typical with prostate cancer. It's very silent. You don't see it. It's hidden wherever in your body it is. In any event, my family doctor recommended I see a urologist. He started with the normal digital [DRE] here in Virginia.

"He didn't notice anything unusual in the digital, but he said, 'Just to be on the safe side I want to do a biopsy.' So he set up for a biopsy, and that is not fun because they shoot needles into your prostate area. He puts a gun in there and pulls the trigger. The needle goes in and takes a sample, and then he comes out and shoots it again. I think it was the day after Christmas when he called me to say I had prostate cancer! It was a 7 on the Gleason scale. I wasn't scared at all. Some people get all scared. But I wasn't. I just asked, 'What are my options?' I said the big thing is I wanna get the thing outta me. My brother left his prostate around. The urologist discussed all my options. Surgery, seed implants, beam radiation. He even offered to send me down to MD Anderson [Cancer Center] in Houston, Texas, where he said he knew the highest-rated radiologist in the country and he was available. He would put in these seeds to kill the prostate cancer. But I told him my brother waited too long and this thing metastasized and he thought radiation would do the job—and he died. I don't want that to happen to me, I told him, 'I want the cancer out!'"

Pat Robertson's urologist was a surgeon. "He said, 'Well, there's something you should know.' He said the problem with radiation is that if the cancer comes back, you've had it! There's nothing else you could do. So then he went on to describe how this radical surgery works. And it sounded like an ungodly mess. You think you'll be incontinent. You think you'll be impotent. But, you know, I trust in the Lord and I decided I wouldn't worry about it. My wife is like I am. I mean, you take what comes around. The doctor took us through the whole procedure, and neither of us was particularly worried. Some people get terribly upset. But I didn't. I knew the Lord was gonna take me through."

Preparation for the surgery began almost immediately. The initial procedure called for Pat to have two units of his own blood drawn and stored in a blood bank a few weeks in advance of the procedure in case blood was needed during his operation. "I was scheduled to go for the surgery on a Wednesday. I wasn't afraid to tell people about it. I didn't want to make a big deal about it if I had prostate cancer. When I mentioned all this to one of my coworkers, he told me to hold on. He said he had just been in touch with a guy who found a doctor in Miami who does laparoscopic surgery on the prostate. And he said this guy was up in about a week after the surgery and was doing fine. I said that sounds interesting."

Pat thought about meeting that surgeon in person and decided to fly down to Miami. "I was immediately impressed with him. I learned that he was very skillful and competent and had studied laparoscopic prostate cancer techniques in France. He had a degree from Columbia, and at the same time, he was a very nice fella. We discussed the laparoscopic surgery procedure, and I finally said, 'When can we do it?' And he asked if I would like to come in the following Monday. I said, 'Okay. You got a deal. Just make the reservation and I'm on the way.'"

Pat says he listened carefully to all the details the laparoscopic surgeon had to tell him. "He showed me a number of people who had had it done and the successes, and he had quite a list of patients on whom he had performed the procedure. I was ready. I'm a risk taker and I've always been a risk taker. The alternative [open radical surgery] sounded so horrible. During our initial talk, the doctor suggested that in the open radical procedure it was like cutting into your gut and flying blind with no lights. Well, that struck me as a horrible procedure. The standard radical sounded awful. That about convinced me to do the laparoscopic. The scrub team was excellent. The anesthesiologist was also a cardiologist. His nurses have been working with him for some time. And I just felt real confident that my surgeon knew exactly what he was doing."

Pat describes the procedure. "They use a gas to inflate your stomach and then they drill a couple of holes and put cameras in so they can see things. And then they drill three or four holes and then send the robot in, and they're able to cut the prostate loose. Then they rejoin the urethra to the bladder. They have to put a catheter in that—kind of a plug to keep it together—and it's about a five-hour operation. Much longer than the open operation. You know, I was walking after a couple of days! I was back on television in seven days and I was riding a horse ten days afterwards! I told my surgeon that I was setting records from surgery to dressage in just ten days! As I say, I was back on my feet the very next day after surgery. I think I spent the night in the hospital, but I was up and around the next day. And then three or four days later, the doctor came by to see me and he said, 'There were no stitches so I'll pull off the Band-Aids.' Let me tell you about the incontinence deal. What I didn't like at all was the catheter. That was the most uncomfortable thing with the whole business. You expect a little incontinence right after the operation and you're hooked up to that catheter. By the end of the week, I was back on television. And surprisingly I was completely dry in just a couple of weeks. As for the potency issue, the doctor couldn't save my nerve bundle. It had cancer in it. True, the libido is kinda gone. I know it takes away a certain amount of pleasure and you feel like you're missing a little something in life. There's no question about it. But it's not a tragedy. My wife and I joke about it. It's so important to have a wife who is supportive. My wife was there with me during the entire time. She's always been very sympathetic. She's a nurse and most nurses are like that. I'm just fortunate to have her. Same goes for my family.

"If you are diagnosed with prostate cancer, I think the biggest thing is not to be afraid of it. And the second thing in my opinion is not to temporize with it. Don't play with it. Get rid of it! It is an evil thing that can destroy you. You can just look around and hope it goes away. It may and it may not. In my opinion, just deal with it first. I found it was the best thing I could do. My message to anybody who has a close male relative in the family—a father, a brother, an uncle—who had prostate cancer is to be tested. A lot of young men think they're not old enough to be tested. Testing only takes a bit of blood and it doesn't hurt. But it can save your life! And then get through it, get a good horse, get on, and ride off into the sunset!"

The Doctor's Notebook

Pat Robertson has confirmed the truth of prostate cancer. It does claim lives, as it did that of his brother. He tells a message that prostate cancer is no longer a taboo subject.

In his account, Pat emphasizes his mission to have his prostate removed after learning of his diagnosis. He was not enthusiastic about the alternative of radiation therapy, and perhaps his brother's experience colored his perspective. However, surgery and radiation are valid alternatives to address prostate cancer, and we do not know how advanced his brother's cancer had been when he received his treatment. When radiation therapy was provided, it is possible that it may have been too late and his disease had progressed. The true message here is that early diagnosis is key so that any form of localized treatment has the best opportunity to control or cure the disease.

It is pleasing to hear that Pat had such a successful outcome with his surgical management. Some truths need to be told, however, in processing his comments. He applauds the circumstances associated with the laparoscopic technique of radical prostatectomy. Clearly he had a highly expert surgeon involved in his care and did well. However, it must be said that the open surgery is not done blindly, and laparoscopic surgery is not inherently superior. Laparoscopic surgery cannot assess cancer directly, because cancer is only determined on a microscopic basis by the pathologists examining tissue under the microscope. Rather, local cancer spread beyond the prostate may manifest itself with various surgical clues of tissue irregularity, which perhaps along with preoperative variables informing the surgeon about the extent of disease would then prompt the surgeon to carry out a more wide resection beyond the immediate borders of the prostate appropriately, irrespective of the surgical approach. The key concept is that expertly performed surgery of any variety in current times yields an excellent result. Patients should expect that in expert hands at a highly experienced medical facility where this surgery is regularly performed, they in general should have low complication rates, rapid recovery, and resumption of normal activities all at about the same rate. Truth be told, anesthesia delivery improvements, overall raised surgical proficiency, and efficient postoperative management have been the principal factors leading to the best outcomes in all patients in the current era.

15

Charles Brickell and Karen Brickell

Sometimes There Are More Questions Than Answers and Nothing Seems to Add Up

Charles Brickell started in construction in 1958, eventually became a painter, and continued in that trade until his retirement in 2002. His wife, Karen, an administrative assistant in the local power company, retired shortly afterward. Charles is a heavyset man with a gentle disposition and easy manner. He and Karen live in a modest white house with blue shutters in Waldorf, Maryland, less than an hour's drive from Washington. These days the Brickells are enjoying life traveling about the country and say they have so far managed to visit just about all fifty states. At the time of this interview Charles was sixty-five, and Karen was sixty-three.

Charles was not into getting annual physicals until he turned fifty-five (in 1998), when his wife insisted he begin. He says he had not a clue what a prostate was and had no recognizable symptoms of trouble until his doctor told him his PSA had come back 4.1 and sent him on to a urologist at a local hospital. "The urologist looked at the report and suggested that I have my prostate removed as soon as possible!

"The thing is, I felt fine. I felt fine all my life until this prostate problem. There was one thing . . . it's hard to explain. But I had this slow pressure urinating. I didn't wake up in the middle of the night to go—or anything like that. It would just take me a little time. I didn't find it alarming. But I didn't think I had any problem.

"When the doctor told me I should have surgery, I have to say I was shocked. But it affected my wife more than it did me. I think I wasn't aware of what I was dealing with. When I heard the words 'prostate cancer,' I started to find out more about it. That's when I stayed in bed—probably like everybody who's been told he has cancer—and you start thinking about it and it bothers you. You kinda keep it inside of you. I didn't think of it as a death sentence. All my life I've dealt with things as they've come along. Ain't no use worrying about it too much because there's nothing you could do about it."

Charles would not simply move ahead and follow the doctor's advice. He said he just felt drained and unmotivated. He confessed to doing nothing. "The urologist I had probably wasn't top of the line. Let's put it like that. I've never trusted doctors too much.

"I just felt I didn't want to know a whole lot. I thought all that will happen is that I'll wind up with too many conflicting points of view. And I kept leaning toward wait and see [expectant management]."

The Brickells have two sons, and one son, Mark, insisted that his dad get a second opinion. He himself was a fan of Johns Hopkins. "At my son's and wife's insistence, I went to Johns Hopkins and met with Dr. Burnett. The Johns Hopkins lab looked at the same slides the local urologist's lab looked at and said they disagreed with their findings. I did *not* have prostate cancer. *Did not at all!* I was really relieved! So everything was going then on the back burner. I was going to go along with my life, saying, well, Johns Hopkins, the best hospital going, couldn't make a mistake. So from 1998 to 2006, I was okay! I told Dr. Burnett I made the decision to wait and see how things went along. If the cancer progressed, I would have the surgery. If it stayed the way it is now, I would just take biopsies every year and see."

Not long after Charles left Johns Hopkins, he began experiencing what he described as an occasional odd feeling in his pelvic area. "It just felt like I had an orange or something down there, just above the penis. I could feel the pressure like there's something down there that's too big. That's the only way I can describe it. Dr. Burnett examined me and said my prostate was very large, and he performed a TURP procedure (transurethral resection of the prostate) for BPH, to remove tiny fragments of tissue through the urethra]. That helped a lot. Ever since, I've had no flow problems. And I don't seem to be having that feeling like there's an orange down there now, but still I do realize my prostate is enlarged. And I am taking medication for that."

Karen Brickell says she can never forget that day in 1998 when she came home from work and Charles was standing there and broke the news she never wanted to hear. "'I have cancer,' he said. I was *totally* devastated. I fell on the floor. Charlie had to help me up and hold me. I was totally out of it. A month later we were at Johns Hopkins for a second opinion. We said let's go for the best, and that's when we found Dr. Burnett, and we loved him. I was scared to death that Charlie was going to die. The word 'cancer'! I thought of my father. He had died of colon cancer."

Dr. Burnett's considered opinion was that there was no need to rush in to remove the prostate. Charles was elated and relieved. But the same news had a different effect on Karen. She sensed the hopefulness in the doctor's words, but at the same time felt uncomfortable and confused. She wondered why two or more doctors could look at the same condition and come up with different opinions about how to proceed. One could say treat it. Another could say don't. Charlie went with his gut. "When you get a second opinion, you can run into the problem where an accredited doctor at one university hospital tells you to 'wait and see' and another doctor at another accredited university hospital says, 'Get it out right away.' What do you do? You pick the one you want to go with, and I picked Dr. Burnett."

Karen said, "So the Hopkins people told us that Charlie did *not* have cancer. The biopsies were negative. For eight years, Charlie continued to show no cancer. Until 2006, when the Gleason was reported to be 6! Those eight years that went by, I just began wondering if Hopkins was right when they first said Charlie had no cancer. My question was, 'Did the local hospital we first went to really make a mistake?' I don't know. I don't know."

In September 2007, Johns Hopkins took another biopsy, and Dr. Burnett still said it showed that though the cancer might still be there, it was not growing. Karen remained uneasy and wanted more reassurance, so they went for a third opinion at another university hospital. The urologist there suggested surgery, and Charles had had enough. He was returning to Hopkins. Karen said, "I just want him to be alive. That's all I care about." And they were back under Dr. Burnett's care. "I once said to Dr. Burnett, 'What is it that I'm not asking you that you need to tell me?' He could hear in my voice and see in my expression that I wanted more than he was giving me. I still feel strongly he should tell us what to do. Why don't two doctors with equal training come to the same conclusions? Just what is it that they are disagreeing on?"

Charles finally put his and his wife's conflicts to rest. He would stick with expectant management. His advice to others: Don't take the first opinion. Go for a second. "I guess it's to be seen whether I made the right decision or not, and somebody else might make a different one. Dr. Burnett promises me that by doing what I'm doing, prostate cancer won't jump up and bite me, just as long as I have PSAs on a regular basis and biopsies, and so far I've had five." In the end, Karen left her demons behind. "I have faith in God. That's who I went to. That's how I got through it. Through my faith, and also it came from Charlie saying, 'All right, let's take one step at a time.'"

Update as of August 2009: Charles Brickell continued the course of expectant management, but in November 2008 his Gleason reading rose to 9. In consultation with his wife, Karen, and Dr. Burnett, Charles elected to have a radical prostatectomy. His surgery was performed immediately after Thanksgiving 2008. Following the operation he was doing well, and his prognosis for a complete recovery is said to be excellent. His case illustrates that expectant management surveillance can pinpoint how and when a patient's minimal cancer has grown sufficiently aggressive for him to consider an appropriate course of treatment.

The Doctor's Notebook

The Brickells tell a story that is rather common. Charles carried a prostate cancer diagnosis, but its threat to claim his life was very low and tough decisions lay ahead with regard to the best way to manage it. Since the late 1980s, men have frequently been getting prostate biopsies because of slight elevations in their PSA values, with the result showing minimal findings of prostate cancer. It should be made clear that Charles's prostate biopsy result initially showed prostate cancer upon pathologic verification at the Johns Hopkins Hospital, not that there was no evidence of prostate cancer. Precisely, the findings revealed prostate cancer that was minimal in extent and aggressiveness such that it represented a low-profile presentation of cancer.

Prior to the availability of PSA testing, prostate biopsies were prompted only by abnormal findings on digital rectal examination, and if cancer was found of any extent, it was thought to be clinically significant as a threat to a man's life. Nowadays, we frequently identify low-profile prostate cancer, which presents a dilemma since much of this may never progress to claim a man's life. Indeed, the Brickells express the common emotional distress of many patients, which is the difficulty of coping with their prostate cancer diagnosis and deferring recommendations regarding management. We urologists also agonize with this diagnosis.

Truthfully, more than 50 percent of men above the age of sixty may carry minimal findings of prostate cancer, and many may die *with* the disease and not *from* the disease. When a man is diagnosed with low-profile prostate cancer (determined by specific pathologic criteria), approaches for management may range from active treatment to active surveillance, consisting of regularly scheduled digital rectal examinations, PSA testing, and prostate biopsies (expectant management). In time, approximately one in four men may declare himself by clinical and pathologic findings to have a prostate cancer that we strongly acknowledge could be a threat to his life and certainly then would demand active treatment.

This dilemma of low-profile prostate cancer, once diagnosed, does permit expectant management. However, the decision to proceed with expectant management or more definitively with prostate cancer surgery or radiation calls for a joint decision between the urologist and the patient and his family. Indeed, risks of active treatment could include erectile dysfunction, urinary incontinence, and others. For some, the risks of the interventions may exceed the threat of the disease. Unfortunately, this is a tough call for us physicians to make. My advice to patients is that if they feel strongly about the threat of the prostate cancer, even if it is defined to our best ability as low-profile, then the patient should indeed proceed ahead aggressively. In my counseling the Brickells, I presented a very straightforward, balanced discussion of all of the issues. Evidently, there was some conflict between Charles and his wife, and I believe he did not want to encounter risks of intervention unless it was clear that he had a truly life-threatening situation. He certainly seemed very calm in electing the option of expectant management.

It is important to comment on Charles's appreciation of pelvic discomfort and changes in his urinary function. His urologic condition included the simultaneous presence of BPH (prostate enlargement) associated with lower urinary tract symptoms (LUTS). This is a benign situation, and it had no bearing on his prostate cancer diagnosis. We addressed his BPH/LUTS as a separate condition, and he clinically improved from a minor procedure. It is important to distinguish the conditions of prostate cancer, which in early stages generally lacks a symptomatic presentation, and BPH/LUTS, which can be symptomatic.

Having cared for the Brickells over many years, I too had developed a special bond with them. Our close relationship was built on trust and my encouragement that they take an active role in becoming as informed as possible about the dilemmas of prostate cancer management. I can appreciate many patients' perspective that we are not giving them some important information or course of action when they are looking toward us for definitive answers. It is not our intention at all to hide anything. Rather, there are situations in the practice of medicine in which limitations exist in knowing the best treatment or predicting disease outcome. It is hoped that with further discoveries we can become more certain in making helpful clinical recommendations.

The terms "watchful waiting" and "wait and see" (sometimes used interchangeably) meant that the patient elected not to have treatment but would wait to see whether cancer developed or became more aggressive. Today, doctors use the term "expectant management." In this instance, doctors take a proactive course of surveillance in following the patient, providing periodic check-ups. These may include PSAs, DREs, and biopsies to determine whether aggressive cancer has developed.

16

Lennox Graham

Does "Minimal Prostate Cancer" Guarantee You a Free Pass?

Lennox Graham is the director of outreach programs at the University of Maryland in Baltimore. He was born in Guyana and came to the United States in 1979 to study plant and soil sciences at Tuskegee University and received a graduate degree in genetic engineering at Ohio State. He came to Baltimore to work as a geneticist at the University of Maryland. His ardent interest in the health issues of African Americans drew him to participate in outreach programs at the University of Maryland and eventually motivated him to focus on helping African American men deal with prostate cancer. Lennox, who often goes by the name "Mr. G," and his wife, Avis, live in Pikesville, Maryland. He was fifty-three at the time of this interview.

Lennox arrived in Tuskegee, Alabama, seven years after news of the notorious Tuskegee Syphilis Experiment broke in the *Washington Star*. That the government deliberately allowed a group of black men suffering from syphilis to die for the sake of an ill-conceived experiment had a stark effect on the country. Among African Americans, it produced mistrust of the government and of white society in general. It had a particularly devastating effect on the student body at Tuskegee University, some of whose officials had assisted the U.S. Public Health Service in carrying out the experiments. Lennox says many in the African American communities have never forgiven the government for what was done. "People do not like the idea of being experimented on. And that is one of the major factors why African Americans shy away from having anything to do with the medical system. As a matter of fact, after the Tuskegee affair, they came to distrust hospitals. They talked about black vans that would come around and snatch up local residents. When some parents discipline their children, they might tell them, 'I'm going to let that van come and get you.' Generation after generation was brought up on this type of fear. They still feel that way, and it is something we have to change."

Lennox Graham did not choose to focus on prostate cancer in the university's outreach program as a result of having the disease himself. His own battle with prostate cancer turned out to be a case of pure irony. "I have a passion for helping people, and I have a passion for dealing with the high incidence of diseases in African American men. That's what really prompted me. I looked at all the diseases—high blood pressure, diabetes, prostate cancer—impinging on black men, and I decided prostate cancer needed my full attention."

Like so many prostate cancer patients, Lennox had no clue that he was about to deal with an insidious and surreptitious foe. He was then fifty-one. "One day I had a strange feeling in my abdomen. It was hard to describe. Not painful but 'funny.' Just a feeling that told me something in that area was not right. I pay very careful attention to my feelings and I decided to take action. I decided to go to my primary care physician and have it checked out. He indicated that it was probably inflammation of the prostate gland. And he gave me some antibiotics to take care of it. But the feeling came back. And I told my doctor, 'Something is amiss here.' And because of my knowledge of prostate cancer, I know the only way you can know for sure if you have prostate cancer is to have a biopsy. That's the true way to know and there is no other answer. He went along with my thinking and gave me a referral. I went to a urologist at the University of Maryland and the doctor performed a biopsy. It was a very embarrassing thing.

Very embarrassing because I felt it would just be the doctor and me in the room. But you had nurses walking back and forth. It was very embarrassing to me. Your feet are in these stirrups, and you're just spread open like that. And people I see every day just walking in and looking at me. It was very, very embarrassing to me. Anyhow, the doctor numbed the prostate area and then went through the anus and he did his random clips of the prostate. There was a little blood in the urine as I tried to urinate. But all in all, it went well. But thanks to God, I went home and the blood left my urine and everything seemed fine.

"About three or four days after that I was in a video conference at work, and I was called out of the room to take a phone call. It was the urologist. He said, 'You have prostate cancer. What you need to do is come and let's get this thing out.' I said, 'What! You know, I'm in a meeting right now, and you give me this type of information on the phone. By myself. Where are the ethics here?' He apologized, but I was shook up for the rest of the day." Lennox was angry. "There was no discussion. No options offered, just let's do the surgery. I sat in my chair for a long while, just contemplating what I just heard. I thought about the people who don't have the knowledge I do and who don't know there are options. They depend on doctors to make decisions for them. Where would someone be who had to depend on a doctor and not be able to make his own determination? Where would that person be today? Some doctors aren't caring enough to give you what you need and when you need it. And many African Americans go to the doctor too late, when the cancer has metastasized. That is a major problem! The irony of it all was, here I am, someone who has been advocating about prostate cancer, and I find myself in the same situation. I am realizing, too, that I know of no one in my family who had died of prostate cancer. I never knew what my grandfather died of. Someone may have died of it but it wasn't to my knowledge.

"Well, my wife and I made an appointment to visit this urologist who called me. He said he can do the operation. He has a neighbor he did the operation on. The man is doing well . . . on and on. Then he began to berate the doctors at Hopkins and said they only operate on the opulent. I would like to say that any time you meet a doctor who is putting down other doctors, that should be a red flag. His actions and remarks were not sitting well with me. He said set your appointment and I'll do the operation. As we were driving home, my wife said something very poignant to me— and it still sticks in my mind. She said, 'I do not have a relationship with your prostate. I have a relationship with *you!*' And I am thankful, and men ought to be thankful, for wives who are caring and understanding of the situation. That was so touching to me. Then she went on, 'I just want you to be here, and that's what's important to me.' Right there and then I decided I was going to do this operation—but this particular doctor would *not* do the operation."

Results of the biopsy taken at the University of Maryland indicated that Lennox had 15 percent cancer cells in only one of the twelve cores taken. "I was having no symptoms and I decided to shop around [for a doctor]. My boss at the University of Maryland, a renowned doctor, advised me to get a second opinion at Johns Hopkins. So I went to Hopkins, met with Dr. Burnett, and immediately felt very comfortable. He was a very positive man, and the first thing he said was that with fifteen percent we don't operate. We are going to do expectant management. My wife and I were very happy to hear that we don't have to have the surgery. We were so happy, so pleased. Then, about a week later, I got a call from Dr. Burnett. He said the pathology lab at Hopkins reviewed the slide and that eighty-five percent of the cells were cancerous! And he said he had now decided to take a more aggressive approach than we had discussed. There was silence on the phone. Dead silence. I was in shock! To think that you had two pathologists—and that one could be so wrong! It just goes to show that this is not a perfect science. Dr. Burnett said I didn't have to make a decision right now. We can talk about it a little later on. Right there I said to him, 'Let's get the operation done.' The truth is that some pathologists have more experienced eyes and can see a different picture of the cells, while others may not recognize the complex morphological differentiations of those same cells.

"I remember I went home and walked into my living room. I sat down and began looking around my house. I was actually coming face-to-face with my own mortality. I said out loud, 'I can actually die!' I'm looking around at my wife's pictures and my children's.

I'm overwhelmed by how fleeting life can be. Everything took on a new meaning for me. Everything looked so special. The trees looked different. Their leaves looked different. It was just beautiful, beautiful. I saw things that I had passed on the road. Never paid any attention to them. Everything looked different that day. And later, when I was traveling down to Hopkins to do the operation, I just felt like telling everybody, 'How are you? How y'doin'?' I just wanted to talk to everybody!

"On November 23, 2003, I checked into the hospital. My pastor came. A strange feeling came over me. I can still remember. We were there together because I knew there was going to be a time in my life that I will not know. I will not ever be able to recall. That's the time when I will go under anesthesia. That's the time when I will not be in control. And that's the time when I realized, what is man? There must be something higher. A higher power. In my case, as a Christian, I knew that God is in control, and *we* are not in control. And so I prepared myself for going up to the operating room. We prayed there. Then I had to make a decision as to whether I wanted a lumbar injection [spinal anesthesia] or to go under with full anesthesia. I opted for the lumbar 'punch' injection. And so I was taken into the operating room. The nurses were so kind, and the doctor indicated he was going to put something into my saline line. All I knew I was sitting up there talking to the nurses . . . and I knew nothing after that. Then, I remember, when I came around in the recovery room, my wife was there and I couldn't move my toes! I was scared as hell. I had the will, but I couldn't move my toes! I'm someone who likes to be in control. With all the willpower I had, I still couldn't move my toes. I had to be patient because after a while I *was* able to wiggle my toes.

"The next day I was up and out of bed. Walking down the hospital corridor with a lot of other men. We called it our little highway. It's times like this you realize how little material things mean, how much just being alive is what counts. The gentleman in the next bed told me he was just forty-two years old, and his PSA was over 24. We talked and developed a bond, and we shared, and I was wondering what was next. I was in so much pain. And he told me the next day I'd be walking without this pain. He was right. Magically, like clockwork, the next day I was walking without the pain. Each day I became stronger. I started encouraging other men who had just come in. Because I was getting ready to leave, and I could see them doing their rounds. And I'd say, 'You gonna do better each day,' and we would just have a ball. We had a bonding. The nurses were so kind to me and took care of me. It was just a wonderful, wonderful experience."

Following his recovery from the prostatectomy, Lennox returned his attention to helping less fortunate men in the black community with prostate cancer. "My role is to help African American men understand how they must stand up to the disease. To help the black community understand how to apply science to improve the quality of their lives. We do workshops in the community that are health-related. We teach people in the community about blood pressure, about diabetes, and I specialize in the area of prostate cancer. Much of the work is through churches and community groups. My word to African American men is this: You can't expect people to give you everything. You must have a burning desire within yourself to want to know and to want to live. Opportunity comes clothed in everyday garments. It's all around you. If you don't have a focus, if you don't have a goal, you'll never realize the things around you."

Update as of September 2009: Lennox Graham says he is completely dry and is doing just fine sexually. He currently teaches global health at Howard University in Washington, D.C.

The Doctor's Notebook

Quite obviously, Lennox Graham has a personal knowledge and passion regarding the condition of prostate cancer. He stresses the importance of early detection and diagnosis of this disease, which by his own experience translates into the best opportunity with treatment to achieve a successful outcome. Because of the early presentation of his disease, he was an optimal candidate to undergo a "nerve-sparing" modification of radical prostatectomy. His case is a very good example of what can be achieved with early diagnosis—cure with preservation of pelvic functions. He effectively communicates how confronting the disease early can be both life-saving and quality of life–saving. He champions this concept for all men, while keeping a special focus on those with a particularly high risk for the disease, African American men.

A teaching point is worth discussing here. Lennox had presented with what appeared to be low-profile disease on the basis of no suspicious findings for prostate cancer on a digital rectal examination and a biopsy result that showed low- to intermediate-grade disease (Gleason score 6) in only 15 percent of one of twelve biopsy cores. Only after his prostate biopsy material was reevaluated was it clear that more disease was present, because the biopsy core showing cancer actually contained 85 percent cancerous cells. The initial pathological interpretation revealed minimal enough and low-threat disease that presented a quandary. The initial findings suggested a presentation that might not ever progress. I had put forward the option of expectant management in this light initially. However, upon further review, the biopsy findings definitely directed a definitive reaction to his disease.

I think it is appropriate to communicate to patients truthfully about their disease state and inform them that we urologists struggle at times to know the exact risk of the disease presentation when only minimal findings are identified. The critical issue in this context is whether the risk of the intervention exceeds the threat of the disease. I ask patients to help me decide how they wish to proceed when this situation arises. This is not meant to suggest that I avoid giving them proper direction or fail to help them with deciding what action they should take. Rather, it is an effort to treat patients as thinking individuals who should partner with me in providing their very best care. It is our practice at the Johns Hopkins Hospital to have outside pathology material rereviewed in our pathology department. More important, we want to do our own "homework" when giving patients the very best of a second opinion. Upon rereview, it was apparent that a greater extent of disease was evident than what was initially reported. The rereview clearly indicated that his cancer presentation was not clinically insignificant. I impressed upon him under this circumstance that definitive management should be pursued without delay. After discussion of treatment alternatives, a decision was made jointly to proceed with radical prostatectomy.

PART IV

Aftereffects

17

Jim S.

When Libido Takes Control

Jim S. was an undercover narcotics cop attached to the Upper Darby, Pennsylvania, Police Department. His rank was sergeant, and we spoke with him in January 2006, shortly after he turned sixty and decided to take retirement. For reasons of security, he prefers to be known here simply as Jim.

"Most of the time I did buys. Collected intel. I worked in plainclothes. I'd go around to bars and houses and did buys on people. Trying to cobble together a case that eventually the drug task force could use and get indictments on. Once you get the technique needed for the law, it's not very tough mentally. You have to be a good actor. By that I mean you need nerve to go into bars and be solicited to buy drugs. Many people can't do it. They're too nervous, give themselves away. People who didn't know me were anxious to sell me drugs. You don't necessarily have to reach out to these people; they'll find you!"

Jim is a heavyset, youthful-looking man, a little over six feet tall. His dark brown hair is now beginning to show specks of gray. He is soft-spoken with a distinctive Philadelphia accent. He graduated from St. Joseph's University and is obviously highly intelligent with the necessary street smarts. Jim is single. He had been married, but after twelve years together he and his wife split up. They had no children. "I was running on her left and right. Cheating on her left and right. And she was just nice enough at the time. I had just bought a new Nissan Maxima. Our settlement was I got the house and she got the car. That was it. She was a nurse and was okay because she was making plenty of money."

Jim says his whole life centered on sex. His job, hanging around bars, gave him constant access to women "My entire life has been a veneer. I consider myself more intelligent than my peers. But I have to say that whatever intellectual life I had did not support me. 'My car is better than yours.' 'Look at all these girlfriends I have at fifty-something years old.' 'Look at all I can do.' 'Look at this cool job I have.' I always tried to keep in shape. I didn't want a big stomach so I'd run a lot and I'd walk a lot. That was to attract women." Jim is an extremely likable and personable man, somebody whose company you'd easily enjoy, and many women he met did. "Sex was always a big part of my life. My life was work, nice clothes, making fun of other people, and seeing how many girls liked me. That was who and what I was. I didn't have an intellectual life to fall back on. I don't know why, because I read everything, and after all, I'm a college graduate.

"I was on the police department wage committee. They wanted to switch health coverage over from Blue Cross to an HMO. So they sent me to find out how many guys had health problems. As part of the process, I had to go to my own doctor to get a signed letter about my health records to turn in to my department. When I dropped in to see my doctor, he asked did I ever have a PSA. Yada, yada, yada. I took the blood test and didn't think much about it. Until I finally had to call him back and ask him about the letter. Almost three weeks had gone by. He said, 'Oh, man, I have to talk to you.'

"He says, 'Your PSA is way up there—46.5!' My doc is a professor of medicine at Jefferson Medical School in Philly. I asked him what that meant. He says, 'It means it's something you can't ignore. Jim, I have to tell you. You have prostate cancer.' I was stunned. I went home and I just sat down. For the first couple of hours, I just sat in that chair. I couldn't concentrate. The first thing that came to my mind was I'm going to die. I mean, I am going to die! Everything just went racing through my mind. I remembered my father had prostate cancer. He was sixty-five, but he didn't die of it. He went on living until he was seventy-seven. And when I started to settle down I remembered people saying if you get to be seventy you're likely gonna have cancer in your prostate, but you'll probably die of something else. Like a truck can hit you first. I didn't know much about the prostate. I knew you could get an enlarged prostate and you could urinate a lot. But I figured you don't have to worry about that until you're older. But I certainly wasn't expecting this kind of news, and I figured it's not something you can just discuss with the guys. You know, the guys I worked with were cops, and cops don't talk about things like that. I certainly didn't. Until it was absolutely diagnosed. I didn't tell anybody I know about it. Then I got switched to a different platoon. I had to tell my lieutenant. Then I told one personal friend. He's seventy-one now and he's dying. He looked after me before and after my operation, and I'm looking after him now.

"Right after I got my bearings, I decided to make appointments with urologists. I actually made appointments with three urologists. I wanted to find out for sure. I kept telling myself, well, maybe it's some mistake. So I went to see these three guys in one week. They all did the same thing. They all did a digital exam. No one ordered a second PSA! And they all came back with the same result. They told me I had prostate cancer!

"Finally, I went online. That's where I found out about the Johns Hopkins Brady Urological Institute. And that's where I decided to go. I went to see Dr. Burnett. He did his little digital exam and said, 'Listen, here's the deal. You are on the cusp of whether we can operate or not. I would say operate. But you should know going in that I have a twenty-five percent chance of getting the whole thing.' That's a twenty-five percent chance he could get all of the cancer. But I said to him, 'That's a seventy-five percent chance that you won't.' I realized that if we didn't go for it, it meant a hundred percent chance that he won't get any of it and I'd have no shot at all! That's when he gave me the really bad news. He said, 'If I get that prostate out, I'm gonna have to get those nerve bundles on either side. So that means no erections till maybe we shoot something up there.' Whatever! Well, that's a tough decision, but if I didn't do it, where would I be now?

"So I went down finally and had the surgery. But I didn't realize that my operation would turn out to be as horrendous as it did. I understand the surgeons were saying mine was one of the most difficult surgeries they'd had to do. After they inserted a catheter in me, I had trouble walking. Fourteen days, and it nearly drove me crazy. Until they took it out! Then—no problem. No problem at all. Then it was a question of how was my PSAs? It would take three months to know the number.

"Next thing I had to deal with was urinary incontinence. That was the biggest shock of all. I remember Dr. Burnett made a production about incontinence. 'You know,' he said, 'our rate of incontinence here is the lowest in the country. It's our trademark basically.' He's talking about wet and dry. In my mind, I'm thinking, am I ever going to have sex again? At that point, I had no idea how big a deal wet and dry was. What a big issue that was. How it was really *the* issue. The thing [catheter] comes out and—well, I've always had a thing with doctors. I never asked them more than I wanted to know. I will take what they tell me, right? I'll never say, 'What happens next?' So, the thing comes out. And I went out to my car with no pad, no nothing. First thing you know I'm saturated! It never dawned on me that I had to wear a pad. Otherwise I'd be soaking wet, right?

"Then it became a question of Kegel exercises [that strengthen the sphincter muscles controlling urination]. Do them, you'll be fine. That's the prescription. I went back a couple of months later for the first PSA. That was good. Zero! Two months after that, I'm back. Dr. Burnett asks how dry I am. I said I'm down to three pads. Another three months I'm back for another PSA. Still good. But I tell Dr. Burnett I'm down to two pads. He gave me some medication to control the urination. It's supposed to squeeze the urethra . . . dry it up a bit—just like Sudafed does. But it didn't work. I'm still leaking and on two pads. And I swear to God, nobody did more Kegels than me. The odd thing was that I could urinate and stop on a dime. Start and stop, just like that. Why was I still not dry? Still having to use two pads. For sure, I was paying the price for finding I had prostate cancer too late!

"Dr. Burnett comes up with a new solution. He says, 'You need an artificial sphincter.' That was the first thing out of his mouth. Some guys just do. I'm guessing that it's a factor that when they do the operation, they may have to take out more tissue than they'd like to. Yet he expected me to be dry and I wasn't. So, I had that sphincter put in and—I *was* dry! I was totally dry except when I did some heavy lifting. I use a small liner all the time, just in case. But for the most part, I'm dry—let's say I'm ninety-nine dry and very comfortable with it. The thing's working great. It doesn't bother me. The way it works is you have to grab your scrotum and give a little squeeze and you can urinate. Then it automatically shuts off."

Jim continued to have other issues. "Just before my surgery I was living with a thirty-two-year-old Asian woman. I made sure that when I got back from the hospital that she was out of the house. Why? Because I didn't want somebody living in the house that I couldn't have sex with. I would like companionship, but I will not meet with a woman I can't have sex with. It's odd. It's wrong. There's something almost inhuman about it. But do I want female companionship? I can't say I want to meet anybody new.

"You may be wondering about women from my past. Well, women I've known for a long time . . . and the sexuality that stopped in the past . . . those women who still know me as a friend. I still talk to them. But potential sex partners? No, I avoid that. There's a caveat I go by. There were two women I once had sex with. There's an unwritten code that I would not have sex with them now. With them, sex is *not* expected now. As far as the women I've had sex with more recently, I pushed them away. I keep them at arm's length. I do it deliberately. I feel diminished. It's surreal. Every man likes something about a woman. I miss talking to women. I miss their conversation. I don't want to meet women like this now. I think a woman thinks, 'Why should I be with him? Why not be with a guy I can have a normal sex life with?' So I don't initiate anything. I miss all that. It's also a catastrophic self-image. I'm not Pierce Brosnan, but still . . . A week after my prostatectomy, I went to a drugstore because I needed to buy glasses to read fine print. Just popped up after the operation. That seems to be a harbinger of my body. All of a sudden, I've thought of myself as an old man . . . or a man getting older. At the age of fifty-eight I never thought of age at all. I thought I would never get old. Now, two years later, every day I am feeling more and more like an old man."

Jim's depression worsened when he discovered that months after his prostatectomy, his PSA score began to rise. It climbed from zero to 4. Dr. Burnett advised radiation. Jim went to the Fox Chase Cancer Center near his home in the Philadelphia area. He was put on hormone therapy and radiation. Jim chose not to go to any support groups. "The original plan was to get radiation for thirty days. When I went to Fox, I would go back for a PSA every three months. My doctor there, Dr. Preminger, said, 'Here's the deal. We're gonna give you radiation. And two years on Lupron. And thirty treatments of radiation. Lupron makes your bone density suspect. So every few months we'll check you out.' Last time I saw Preminger, he said, 'We might go past two years with you because your bone density is good. So you may go longer than two years on Lupron.'

"Lupron is a drug they give you when you still have a PSA after they've taken your prostate out. It drops your testosterone to a level that you no longer think about sex or women! It is absolutely the oddest state of being! It *is* surreal. Every man has something about a woman that attracts him. Some like big boobs. Some like other attributes. I like legs. Now it's like a hollow memory of what I used to like. They don't affect me at all. It's an odd way of viewing life. I actively avoid attractive women. I have no interest in them anymore at all. And I know . . . I know this loss of feeling, call it what you like, it has nothing to do with age. Another thing, I sometimes get hot flashes. I don't get that many, maybe one a week. I may be sitting and suddenly I feel hot. Maybe for thirty seconds. When they lower your testosterone—and that's what Lupron does—it raises your estrogen level, and you can get the same symptoms a woman experiences during menopause.

"Maybe my outlook would be different if I had had children. Until now, I never thought about that. But it's possible. Because if you have children, you broaden your horizons to realize that other people's feelings are more important than yours. A person with a family is not going to be fixated on himself."

The encouraging news about Jim is that in June 2006 he reported that his radiation and hormone treatments have been effective and that his PSA score was again back to zero. His spirits were appreciatively higher and he has begun developing new friendships and new interests.

Update as of November 2008: Following Jim's radical prostatectomy in September 2003, he had difficulty adjusting to his post-surgical lifestyle. Over time, he found he could restart his life. He returned to the University of Pennsylvania to begin Arabic studies, and his grades were outstanding. He recaptured a new social life and found new friends and new interests. His mood is now upbeat. Today, he finds himself content, happy, and pleased that his life has taken a new and positive direction. Jim will tell you that his hopes have been realized. His PSA level has remained at zero. In short, Jim has begun life anew.

The Doctor's Notebook

Jim tells a very sobering story. He mentions many of the challenging aspects of having prostate cancer and then undergoing treatment for it. There are realities that his case exemplifies when the patient is diagnosed late and thus has a situation that is tough to manage. His testimonial also is revealing to me with regard to how patients again sense, hear, and understand many aspects of their prostate cancer management.

As I reflect on his case history, several issues resonate with me. It is worth observing that he has had a strong focus on sexual activity and relationships with women. This conceivably is common to many men. Indeed, this aspect of quality of life can be quite important. Unfortunately, it seems that this focus interfered with his attention to his own health. I suspect that he knew prostate cancer could have ramifications with regard to a man's sexual ability, and he was in a state of denial about his potential risk to have the disease. He does acknowledge that prostate cancer was immediately known to him in that a friend and his father had carried the diagnosis. He admits that he had not been very vigilant about his health. A presentation of locally advanced prostate cancer bordering on inoperability along with frankly a very high PSA measurement indeed implied a concerning case presentation of the disease. Eventually, he describes his acceptance of the disease and that it can have an impact on one's way of life. A greater truth may be that along with this experience he came to appreciate that life does bring about changes. He mentions his adaptation to getting older by virtue of having to use eyeglasses for reading.

More profoundly, I believe Jim was grappling with an element of depression amid the consequences of his surgery and the circumstances of his life. I have witnessed depression in many men following prostate cancer treatment, whether they are cured or not. It is interesting that some men experience depression even when complete eradication of their prostate cancer is achieved. I know that the whole experience of having and then undergoing treatment for prostate cancer heavily affects most men. Emotional stress would certainly arise from being dealt this disease state, enduring temporary or permanent bodily function losses following its treatment, or even acknowledging one's own mortality. At a minimum, prostate cancer brings about life changes, among them the realization that we will not forever be young and virile. That is the reality of life. Jim was able to take supportive action and successfully adjusted to his new life.

Other realities associated with his prostate cancer management warrant a word or two from the medical perspective. Jim faced the reality of urinary incontinence following his radical prostatectomy. It is quite likely that the need to excise tissue widely surrounding the prostate to attempt to achieve eradication of his disease had a role in the compromise of his pelvic functions. As surgeons, we constantly agonize over the concept of locally advanced disease as we balance considerations of cancer control with the retention of urinary and sexual functions. In his case, it became apparent that he was not making enough standard, spontaneous progress that many men do in the recovery of their urinary control after undergoing radical prostatectomy surgery. After thoroughly discussing the options, we agreed that inserting an artificial urinary sphincter device would be the proper management plan for him. We proceeded with this intervention and successfully addressed the condition.

Another tough reality was that his cancer recurred. Again, this development reflects the local aggressiveness of his disease. We forthrightly reacted to this situation, examined his alternatives, and then carried out a necessary treatment plan. Some men may require additional treatment with radiation accompanied by male hormone suppression, if their cancer diagnosis requires it. It would be my hope that all men obtain a prostate cancer diagnosis that is early and most amenable to a definitive cure at a time when our interventions can be expected to retain bodily functions.

Perhaps the biggest message to be offered by Jim's story, notwithstanding that treatments exist for treating advanced disease, is that early diagnosis and treatment of prostate cancer are advantageous and always preferred.

18

Bruce Hamlette
Getting Your Sex Life Back

Bruce's Hamlette's voice was deep and robust, but his words were sparse and guarded. From our initial phone conversation I had the impression our conversation in person would be difficult. After all, we would be discussing very personal and intimate issues, and I prepared myself for an awkward interview. When I drove up Hudson Avenue near his condo in Bloomfield, New Jersey, I had no idea which of the many buildings on the right side of the street was his. Off to the left, I could see a large pond filled with ducks. I rang his cell phone for directions. His ringer played a jazz riff, and he answered immediately. "Look up," he said. "Do you see me waving?" And there he was, a tall figure in a cap, waving on a second-story balcony.

He greeted me warmly and led me to his small bachelor's quarters, where we sat down on his comfortable sofa and I began to set up my recorder. He kept his cap on and everything about his bearing and his conversation told me my initial reservations were wrong. Bruce Hamlette and I would have no difficulty talking about his prostate cancer—or anything else!

At our meeting in November 2007, Bruce struck me as a gentle giant, poised, wearing thin-framed glasses, very intelligent, with a lot of fire in his belly. He projects great pride in his African

American heritage, and that is infused in his conversation. He was sixty-one years young. He lives alone in this middle-class suburb of Newark. His comfort zone is his studio pad, small yet stocked with everything he feels he needs. His living room by necessity also serves as a clothes closet. You are careful not to step on any shoes alongside the coffee table or disturb any of the electronic equipment.

Bruce was a special education teacher in the Newark, New Jersey, school system. His students ranged in age from nine to twelve. They were, he says, children with behavioral disorders. His job was to help each child develop awareness and in the process learn how to think and function in society. To do that, he would have to raise them from the total despair that had surrounded their lives since birth, to build hope from the ashes of social and economic catastrophe that had damaged their young lives. It was not and is not an easy job, but Bruce has always viewed his work as a spiritual calling.

If you ask him whether he is retired, he asks you to define retirement. For Bruce, retirement simply means no more paychecks, but his mission itself must go on. Today, he works as a volunteer, carrying on his "salvage operation" for African American youth. He continues to mentor and teach troubled young people at the Essex County Juvenile Detention Center in Newark. Do these tough youths listen to him? "They're tough, but they love me. As a matter of fact, I had one student I saw the other day at the correctional facility. He was so glad to see me, he was telling the other inmates, 'That's my son!' He calls me his son. My experience in special education lets me know that I may have lost a battle, but I have not lost the war!

"When I have a bad day, it prompts me to start thinking about an approach for the next meeting. How to overcome their propensity to look away from their realities. They smile and laugh to keep from crying and they have pride. You have to crack the shell, let them know that it's all right to express their feelings and their anger and their disappointments. Teaching them is a work in progress. It's not something you deal with in two days. It might not click in for three years! I've seen results. When I achieve this, I give all the praise to my Creator. Because He has blessed me to be able to do this, and I feel as though I am a good servant, and though I'm normally struggling, I'm not suffering."

Bruce is divorced and has a grown daughter and two grown sons. He has hypertension and diabetes and on average has been going for medical check-ups every six weeks since he was in his late thirties. In 2000, his primary physician in Paterson, New Jersey, sent him to a urologist, who examined him and said, "You have cancer!" Bruce said the doctor began to laugh and said to Bruce, "Aren't you scared?" Bruce lost his cool. "'No, I ain't scared of a fuckin' thing. Now just hurry up and let me get outta here because I resent your comment.' Maybe he considered his remark humorous. I didn't." Bruce was even angrier after he learned that the urologist had not even sent the biopsy samples out to the lab when he made his pronouncement. Later, when the lab results did come back, Bruce learned that they were negative. The urologist called Bruce's primary doctor, who in turn called to tell Bruce the good news—he was okay!

In 2004, Bruce consulted a new primary physician, who sent him to a second urologist. This doctor performed another series of biopsies and gave him different news. He indeed had prostate cancer, and it was aggressive. His PSA was 14 and his Gleason score was 7! "It's true this urologist offered me the options of radiation or surgery, but he was a surgeon and was pushing for me to get an operation. In any case, he told me, I'd probably need to have a penile implant. But he was just commercial and displayed no humanity or concern about my mental disposition. And to me that made him suspect. I made up my mind that I was not going to let *him* cut me. You have to feel the humanity in the doctors you're dealing with; every doctor is not the same. Like I told my friends, before I just let him cut me, I'm ready to die. But I'm not going to be mutilated like a slave.

"When you get the news that you have prostate cancer, your whole life, what you were going through, and what you were try-ing to achieve . . . the family. . . that whole thing comes across. And then it has a trickle-down effect on you. You gotta be a fighter. You gotta have faith. You cannot allow yourself to sink down into hopelessness. If I was gonna die, it wouldn't be because I turned myself in. You gotta come and get me! 'Cause I'm a fighter. I may not win, but that's how I choose to go out. So then I did my research. Research, research . . . my life was at stake! I made a few more appointments with doctors. And I found out that Johns Hopkins has a reputation for successful treatments and good outcomes for cancer patients."

Initially, he had anxieties and crying spells. But he had two gentlemen friends who treated him royally, including one who took him back and forth to Johns Hopkins. His other friend would go with him too. Both would call him daily to see how he was doing. "When I got to meet Dr. Burnett at Johns Hopkins, I thought God sent him to me. He's the only one I could deal with. His genuineness . . . I would have trusted him for anything he did to me. Dr. Burnett reviewed my case and told me I was too late for surgery. My cancer had advanced too much, and he recommended radiation. I remembered that when I was a little kid my father's brother died of cancer."

Bruce felt the woman in his life for the past eight years would help him get past his agony. He was hurting and craving her warmth and tenderness, and so he told her how much he needed her at this time of his life. "She was a professional woman, an assistant to the superintendent of schools, and when she heard my news, she turned her back on me. She ended our relationship. She said she was not in love with me anymore! She never said, 'I'm leaving you because you got cancer.' She never said that. But I knew that! I didn't know if she or my cancer was killing me. I didn't know which was worse. This apartment, where we are sitting right now, is where I cried, I screamed . . . I rolled over . . . I just dug my fingers into the carpet. I couldn't sleep for days. I couldn't eat.

"Later I told myself it didn't matter. I wasn't concerned with what she figured. I was concerned with what *I* was thinking. You know, the truth comes out in many ways. Some people, they have title and position, and it becomes more important than true love. And I believe in true love. So, it hurt me real bad, but I knew I couldn't ask her to be with me because I'd only be asking for more trouble."

Facing cancer alone is punishment for anyone. Bruce says he has been fortunate in having the support of his children. "When

I told my eighteen-year-old son, I must say he was like my father. He'd be on me. 'Dad, you all right?' He talked to me as though he had this sense of looking after me. This is my younger son. My older boy—when he heard the news, he cried. He loves me, too. That's one of the things that's helped me through, knowing that my children love me unconditionally."

Bruce began his radiation treatment at the Clara Maass Medical Center in Belleville, New Jersey. His doctors prescribed hormone therapy prior to his external beam radiation. "The radiation lasted twenty-eight weeks. I was feeling drained and sore towards the end. Once you get the whole dose, you're very sore, and you have to sit down in a certain way and start being careful.

"At the end of the radiation I found that I couldn't get an erection. Then the doctor said, 'You have aggressive cancer,' and I went along with his suggestion to have seeds. And I took a couple more hormones, and shortly after that, my PSA was down to 0.1. That was maybe two years ago, and the last report I got I was still 0.1!"

Bruce now has yearly check-ups at Johns Hopkins to make certain his cancer has not recurred. At some point following his radiation treatments, he decided to address his inability to have erections. Dr. Burnett performed penile reconstructive surgery and provided him with a penile implant. Bruce spoke about his comfort level with the device and about his progress. "You go through several stages. The first is that you have something foreign in your body. And there's gonna be a period of time where you're gonna have to make the connections psychologically. People wonder if my natural penis was removed. In my case, the answer is no. Dr. Burnett had to reconstruct the penis because the radiation left a lot of scar tissue. And if I hadn't had a penile implant, no one would ever have told me about the scar tissue or the fact that he had to reconstruct my penis. Because he could bend it all the way over to the right. It was broken in a sense. So he had to rebuild it and get all the scar tissue out and then he implanted the device. In just the last month or two, I'm really getting comfortable with how to use it. How to get the erection and how to get some feeling of intimacy and sexuality out of having sex with it. It takes time getting used to it. As for sensation, yes, I do have sensation. The only thing I can't do is ejaculate. But often I get a sensation that feels like an ejaculation. A lot has to do with my mate! The psychology of it all. And you don't get that right away because this is a foreign object in you, and you have to synchronize with it psychologically. When I walk around, I don't even feel anything out of the ordinary. I mean, I don't even know it's there!"

Bruce is a believer in the benefits of adding holistic additives to his diet. "I've always been into the benefits of herbs and vitamins. And I don't think they get the credit they deserve. I believe herbs help me as much as anything else. I don't think they can cure cancer, but I think they can offset it. It's a positive aspect of trying to keep your health up."

What has Bruce Hamlette's experience taught him? "For a few years, I had to go not only without sex but without being able to participate . . . and I withdrew. There was a time when I could look at a woman and not even see her. Then there was a time when I could notice her. Then I had to make a decision. Am I gonna just back up out of life, or am I gonna enjoy myself even if I can't have an erection? So I said to myself, 'This is what I'm gonna do: I'm gonna interact with them. I'm gonna talk junk. I'm just gonna be honest about what I can do and what I can't do. I'm not quitting.' Because it's a major part of life, sex is. But it's not the whole thing. Life doesn't end for you because you can't satisfy a woman sexually. It's your job to try to do the best you can, and it's your job to have the courage and the faith in God to accept where life takes you. But as far as your predicament, you have to take the responsibility of it, and you have to learn and study.

"I would like to say this to other men. Prostate cancer is a pretty big battle and a pretty big pill to swallow. But the quality of life is not in longevity but how you've lived it. I was told a long time ago life is beautiful. You just have to learn how to live it. I think if I should die tomorrow of cancer, I think I went through this thing with determination and I give all praise to my Creator about it. But you must believe. Have faith because your mind and your thinking is as much medicine as any radiation or anything else you're gonna get. Life has no guarantees. It's not the length of time you live, but the quality of life and fulfillment that you have."

The Doctor's Notebook

Bruce Hamlette's story offers several important lessons. Perhaps the most critical lesson is that it illustrates the essential role of a healthy doctor-patient relationship. In Bruce's case, although he was thankful for his treatment outcomes, he suffered consequences because of the delays in the management of his prostate cancer that were directly related to the constrained if not discordant interactions with his personal health advisers and his first-line physicians. It is quite disappointing to me that the confusion and then misdirection regarding his prostate cancer diagnosis led Bruce to lose faith in his physicians, resulting in his setback. Thankfully, Bruce's self-reliance and fortitude enabled him to move forward with the serious issues in his life. Also to be acknowledged is the support of trusted individuals and his religious faith.

Bruce's case also provides an opportunity for me to comment on the management of erectile dysfunction following interventions for prostate cancer. His case reveals that men undergoing prostate cancer treatments do not have to resign themselves to a life without acceptable sexual function. Rather, opportunities exist to restore sexual function and its quality of life associations. Bruce describes a loss of penile erection and a penile deformity that followed his radiation treatments. Acknowledging but not accepting these conditions, he moved forward to seek management advice. I was glad to renew my relationship with Bruce after previously having a serious discussion with him about the missed opportunity for surgical resolution of his prostate cancer. With our reacquaintance, we discussed management options for erectile dysfunction, and he elected to proceed with surgical reconstruction of the penis and then insertion of a penile prosthesis. He did well with this surgery, acknowledging that it has made a difference. Certainly, this additional urological management has allowed him to resume an aspect of his life that was only temporarily lost.

19

Father Ronald Hazuda

His Prayers for a Miracle Find a Response in an Ingenious Device

Father Ronald Hazuda is an Orthodox priest who officiates at St. Nicholas Orthodox Church in Erie, Pennsylvania. In the latter part of 2008, Father Ron celebrated the fiftieth anniversary of his ordination. We spoke with him in January 2008 in Pittsburgh, where he had driven for this interview from his home in Erie. He is a heavyset man with snow white hair and silver-rimmed glasses who is soft-spoken and gracious.

Father Ron's parents emigrated from eastern Europe and settled in a small mining town in the Pocono Mountains region of Pennsylvania, where his father became a coal miner. Father Ron attended Penn State University and Christ the Savior Seminary and completed his studies at Gannon University in Erie. He was seventy-two when we met.

Father Ron is a man with strong family ties. His son, George, runs his own advertising business in Erie. His daughter, Tammy, works for the U.S. Postal Service. In 2006, his family went through three major crises. Dolores Hazuda, Father Ron's wife of forty-seven years, was diagnosed with emphysema and given six months to live. She died on June 30, almost six months to the day from her diagnosis. Tammy's husband, John, developed third-stage esophageal cancer, and surgeons removed his entire esophagus and three-quarters of his stomach to combat his illness. George's wife announced that she had been unfaithful to him and had decided to walk away from their marriage. For Father Ron, it was a threefold crisis. "I lost my wife. My son-in-law, John, with esophageal cancer, was told he had only a few more years. He was only forty-nine. My son, George, was devastated from his broken marriage. I was faced with three terrible tragedies all at once."

Prior to all this, Father Ron learned that two of his brothers had prostate cancer. "My oldest brother didn't want invasive surgery; he elected to have seed implantation. What they failed to tell him was that there were two strengths of seeds—one very aggressive, the other less so. And they gave him the more aggressive. His bladder became perforated, and two years later he fell asleep with the Lord; he died.

"My other brother chose the radical surgery. In two months' time, he was well. He didn't have any severe incontinence. About a week after surgery, he developed a hernia. They repaired the hernia; that was six years ago, and he is doing well today."

Extreme stress finally drove Father Ron to his primary doctor for a complete physical. The doctor discovered that his PSA had gone up from 3.4 to 4.2 within a matter of six months and sent him to a urologist. "I was devastated when the urologist told me that about ten percent of my prostate was cancerous on one side. I felt confused. I just knew that my lifestyle was different from both of my brothers, and I just felt that now there's some truth in that you can inherit cancer. What puzzled me was the fact that my dad never had it. He was a coal miner and had black lung disease. But, surprisingly, my dad died at the age of ninety-one! At age seventy-one, he had a pacemaker put in for an irregular heartbeat, and it worked well for him. My mother was only sixty-six when she died; she had a heart attack and she had had cervical cancer.

"I always tried to take care of myself. I felt I was in tip-top shape. I exercised about an hour every day, religiously, from eleven o'clock to noon. I created my own calisthenics program. I did some walking and weights, I watched what I ate, stayed away from a lot of high-caloric and fatty foods. It was amazing; I had lost forty to fifty pounds. I felt great. In fact, everybody said I was like a new me.

"I met with a young urologist—I'd say in his thirties. He was full of energy. My son, George, was with me. The doctor assured me that everything would be good. I was in good hands. And so I went through all the tests, the stress tests and all the rest at the hospital, and everything came out fine. They told me the Gleason was around 6—borderline, and this doctor felt the prostate should be removed. But then he said, 'If you don't want to do anything right now, we can give you a shot. It's very expensive, but it'll delay everything for about three months.' He said, 'I have a lot of people who do that after they learn that they have prostate cancer.' To be honest, I don't know what kind of shot he gave me, but I can tell you it was very expensive! He made me feel comfortable, but then my primary doctor seemed to have some reservations and said, 'Maybe you should go and get another opinion before you go back to this doctor.' But the thing was I felt comfortable with him. I mean, he assured me that there would be no problems.

"Then when a priest friend of mine in Binghamton, New York, heard I was entertaining getting surgery in Erie, he called me up and said he had done exhaustive research for me on prostate cancer, and he recommended that I go to Johns Hopkins in Baltimore for a second opinion. When I told him I was still planning to have an operation in Erie, he got very upset. He talked to me for maybe half an hour and pleaded with me to go to Baltimore and get that second opinion. I told him I just couldn't in good conscience leave my family because they needed me here in Erie. And I had to put myself last. Later, I learned what a foolish mistake I had made."

Father Ron continued to struggle with his decision whether to go through with the surgery. And which surgery: open radical or robotic? "My wife was gone by now and she couldn't help me. I was living alone and was very stressed out with no one to turn to. It's true the kids came along to the doctors. And they went over everything with me. But it was also true they left the decision to me. They would say, 'If you feel comfortable, then we'll be here for you.' I talked to my primary doctor again, and this time he said, 'I met that urologist socially and I hear he's a very good doctor.' But he started to vacillate and finally said, 'Well, maybe you ought to go to the Cleveland Clinic or someplace like that.'

"My prayer life increased several hundredfold, so to speak. I was praying longer . . . private prayers, you know . . . by myself. My children constantly came by to visit and had me over to their house. They wanted to reinforce that family structure that was so important, and we got strength from each other. My parishioners knew that I was grieving a lot since I lost Dolores. But they also sensed that there was something else bothering me, and so one day I decided to confide in my board. I said I was going through a difficult time and a decision had to be made. I had prostate cancer. I told them it was not in an advanced stage, but I felt that rather than have some chemo, radiation, or some other kind of therapy, I thought I should have it removed."

In late January, Father Ron reached his decision. He would have robotic surgery in Erie. "I went in for the operation on January 26. When I came out of surgery, I was heavily sedated. My children wanted to know why I had been in surgery not for four and a half hours, but for five and a half hours. The doctor told them, 'We ran into a problem. We had difficulty removing the prostate.' He said, 'It had got all chewed up.' Those were his exact words. And then he added, 'But don't worry; everything will be okay.' I was very sick. I was constantly throwing up. I was in tremendous pain, and they wouldn't or couldn't tell us what was wrong. All I knew was that I was very sick. So they gave me a lot of medication to settle me down . . . to eliminate the nausea and the throwing up. Well, I was in the hospital for five days. Finally, they released me from the hospital and sent me to stay with my daughter.

"I stayed with her for a month. I had trouble with my bowels and the incontinence was unbearable. I was even having leaking through the catheter. They were ordering different medications and I had to have visiting nurses. I knew then that I had made a big mistake—never asking this doctor how many of these operations he had done! I was paying the price. I did think about a malpractice suit, but then I said to the children, you know, what are we gonna do? And the reason I said that was because when I went back to this doctor for a check-up and told him I was having all these problems with leakage and everything else, he kept telling me not to worry, everything is going to be okay. That was his response when I told him I was changing pads every hour and a half, around the clock, and that I couldn't sleep more than an hour or two. I had to get up constantly because I was soaking wet, using the heaviest towels I could use.

"Soon afterwards I called him up again, and this time I said, 'You gotta do something because this is getting out of hand.' And that's when he said, 'We'll order you a clamp, a device that fits over the penis and is supposed to put pressure on the urethra.' Well, that didn't work. Finally, I went to my primary doctor, who said, 'This is ridiculous.' He ordered something called a Hollister [a condomlike catheter that amounts to an external collection apparatus that fits over the penis]. You're in effect wearing a condom twenty-four hours. It's supposed to take care of the incontinence temporarily. The Hollister didn't work either.

"I went back to the urologist and said, 'Look, there's something wrong. Everybody else is healing and I'm not.' And he said, 'Let's go in and do a cystoscopic exam again.' He did that, and he says, 'There's some restriction at the mouth of the bladder. Maybe when we sutured it, it was too tight. We'll go back in there and make an incision and try to relieve some of the pressure.' That meant another surgery, and that was May 17. He went through the penis and did that procedure and it didn't accomplish anything, except now I was doing a lot of bleeding. He told me it was from the sutures and I'd be okay. I told him I wasn't okay. And, in fact, the catheter kept getting plugged up from a blood clot. I called the hospital and they told me to force some pressure—pinch the tiny tube from the catheter and maybe I could force the clot through. After two hours I managed to push that clot through."

Desperate for help, Father Ron turned once again to his primary physician, who immediately sent him to the renowned Cleveland Clinic for a second opinion. Once there, Father Ron said the urologist on duty had no solutions to offer. "He refused to look at the medical papers I brought and said, 'I don't want to look at these because the surgeon never puts everything in there that he does in an operation!' We were appalled at this doctor's absolute arrogance.

"I felt I was running out of options and decided I had to have yet another meeting with the urologist who had performed the robotic surgery. Now he came up with the idea of inserting a sling under the sphincter muscle to see if that would help my incontinence. That would require another operation. I realized that he was experimenting with me. I went home and told my children, 'I can't let him touch me anymore.' The hospital sent me a follow-up letter to schedule me, and I called them and said, 'I'm not coming back. I've made up my mind to see someone who is really going to help me.'"

Father Ron's daughter, Tammy, had driven down to Pittsburgh for the interview with him, and she spoke of the emotional trauma that followed her mother's passing. "Right after we lost Mom there was Dad diagnosed with prostate cancer. And just a short while before, his two brothers found they had prostate cancer. In fact, one of them died. I was scared for Dad. It was so painful to watch what he was going through—the aftermath of his surgery and all. Especially when you just think about what a self-sufficient person he'd always been. Suddenly he's having to rely on other people to help him with his problems."

Father Ron says his robotic operation nearly destroyed him. "I couldn't go anywhere. If I tried going somewhere, I had to carry a bag of pads with me. Right after my first operation in Erie, I went to visit a parishioner who was suffering from cerebral palsy. I would go regularly and help him pay his bills. Well, on this one occasion, I finished the work and was ready to leave when I felt a warm gush of urine that ran down into my shoes. I was so embarrassed. I just said to my parishioner, 'George, I gotta go. I just remember some important business I have to take care of.'

"There was another time at church. You know, my church services would run about an hour and a half, and right before services I would put on a new pad, and immediately after church I would go home. I wouldn't go downstairs and socialize because the incontinence was so great. One Sunday morning I was at the altar serving. All of a sudden I felt a severe pain down near the penis area. I was wearing my flowing vestment . . . and then I felt urine gushing down my legs. Nobody noticed it because I was wearing the vestment, but I made a beeline for the side room to change.

I was so embarrassed. I felt I might just have to give up officiating at church service. I mean, I was so stressed out that my primary doctor put me on a pill because he said he was worried about me and I am not the same person he knew last year.

"At about this time, I heard from my priest friend again in Binghamton. That's when he told me that he too had been diagnosed with prostate cancer. And he had gone to Johns Hopkins and was referred to Dr. Arthur Burnett, who did a radical prostatectomy. He said he was now doing very well. Then he told me about a man in the hospital who had had the robotics operation. My friend said he himself was up and out of bed in a day or so, was walking the halls and feeling very good. But the gentleman with the robotic surgery was still in bed—three days after his surgery.

Father Ron says he did not need to hear more. He drove down to Baltimore to see Dr. Burnett. "I was sitting in the waiting room at Johns Hopkins next to a young couple from West Virginia and they told me they had driven all the way to see Dr. Burnett even though they could have gone to Pittsburgh. When they talked to their friends and found out who operated on them and found out their successes, they came to Hopkins."

Dr. Burnett listened quietly and intently as Father Ron related his medical fiasco. At last, he proposed an answer to this seemingly elusive incontinence problem. The solution was an ingenious device called an artificial sphincter. It would involve a minor surgical procedure to insert the device, a six-week healing period, and a second visit to fully activate the device. The sphincter provides a collar that surrounds the urethra and allows the patient to loosen the collar, thereby allowing him to urinate. In about two minutes, the collar automatically closes again, shutting off leakage, not unlike turning off the tap on a sink.

Father Ron had learned a hard lesson. This time before committing himself to the procedure, he carefully did his research and called other patients who had the device implanted to check out its efficacy. When the feedback he needed was positive, then and only then did he consent to the operation.

"I think this experience has been a learning process. I think prostate cancer is not something to keep to yourself or make a decision with one or two people. It should be done with people who are knowledgeable. People who have experienced the same problems you've had."

Update as of November 14, 2009: About two months after Father Ron had his artificial sphincter inserted, I called him to see how he was doing. My phone call interrupted him while he was doing his daily workout. He told me he was doing his routine exercises—bending, stretching, and lifting weights. What he wanted to impress upon me was that he is now able to do all of these exercises without fear of being wet or even dripping. Prior to his sphincter insertion he wasn't able to exercise because of his incredible incontinence.

"Like I told you before," he said, "I am truly a new man!"

The Doctor's Notebook

Father Hazuda shares a touching story. When I first met him, I saw a depressed man with a broken spirit, faced with a daily reminder of the consequences of his prostate cancer treatment. Along with some significant life setbacks, he certainly seemed to have been unfairly dealt many tragedies in life. At the same time, he seemed to be a positive and caring individual, perhaps so much so that he put others' needs above his own. I could see he was a special person, who was in need of receiving help this time.

His story provides a look at the devastation of urinary incontinence that can follow radical prostatectomy. His problem was most severe. The complication had developed following robotic radical prostatectomy, which has been touted as a major advance in the surgical management of clinically localized prostate cancer. However, as this story reveals, surgical complications including urinary incontinence may follow robotic surgery as much as any other surgical approach, and this approach does not obviate any potential risks of this sort. It is important to recognize that the prostate is situated in the pelvis directly adjacent to the male sphincteric complex, and any treatment for prostate cancer, including all varieties of surgical approach, presents potential risks of postoperative urinary incontinence.

I am glad that Father Hazuda came to see me, so that we could move forward with addressing his problem rather than his just accepting it. We were able to have an honest, straightforward conversation about his complication, discuss alternatives for further management, and consider what option would give him the best success in becoming continent. He had already explored lesser invasive options, which were not successful or suitable for him. Other options such as medications would certainly fail given the severity of the condition. A surgical approach seemed appropriate, but I was not in favor of the not always definitive male sling surgery option given the severity of his incontinence. We discussed the option of artificial urinary sphincter device surgery in great detail, covering all potential risks and expectations. I was pleased he was able to carry out further evaluation of this option himself, even speaking with other individuals who had been through this additional surgery. He moved forward with this option, which dramatically changed his life. Once he became continent, he was able to resume his normal life activities, and I was overjoyed to see a man return to his whole self once again.

20

Lloyd T. Bowser Sr. and Dr. Geneva Bowser

Too Little Too Late: The Challenges of Surviving Prostate Cancer

Until his retirement in 1995, Lloyd Bowser was the director of the U.S. Office of Personnel Management, formerly the Civil Service Commission, in Maryland. He was responsible for the enforcement of federal personnel regulations and evaluating agencies' personnel programs and also served as one of Baltimore's commissioners, overseeing the city's Board of Education budget. He is credited with helping to convert the former Orioles and Colts stadium, known today as Stadium Place, into much-prized housing for senior citizens.

Lloyd, a distinguished-looking African American, lives with his wife, Dr. Geneva Bowser, an educator and registered nurse, in a countrylike Baltimore enclave. Neighbors are seen meticulously caring for their gardens and stopping by to visit one another to chat and exchange pleasantries. The streets are pure Norman Rockwell. The Bowsers have three sons. The youngest is a physician, the middle one a podiatrist, and the oldest a computer systems analyst. When Lloyd Bowser told his story in May 2006, he was sixty-seven.

"In 1992, for no apparent reason, I suddenly began losing weight. Sixty pounds! I had always been a person with abundant energy. I was at work often before seven, and I wouldn't leave before five—every day. And then I would go to community meetings on education or other events like my neighborhood association, things like that. It carried me out quite a bit with the very taxing job I had. I began to drag around. I started coming home at four-thirty, which for me was unheard of. I would go into my study in the basement and spend hours there just feeling exhausted. I missed my annual physical, and my wife suggested I see our family doctor. When I went in to see him, he did some blood work on me, which prompted him to call me back. He indicated that I had a PSA of 32! I didn't have a clue what a PSA was. In fact, I didn't know about the prostate or that I even had one. Anyhow, he explained to me what a PSA was and said a normal PSA ranges from 1 to 4 for the majority of men. But for black men the normal PSA can be 0 to 2.5. And mine was 32, so he suggested I see a urologist.

"The urologist did a biopsy. He went in, took seven snippets, and couldn't find any cancer. I was just overjoyed by that. But my PSA jumped to 38 right after the biopsy. And I began to notice that I was having sudden and continuous pain in the rectal area. The pain just began to get worse, so I decided to get a second opinion. I went to the VA Medical Center in Baltimore and asked the physician there if he could do another biopsy. This time the results showed that I had prostate cancer in not one but two of the snippets! I started to ask questions about my family history. I recalled that my dad had had it. But then, he was ninety years of age when he died. What the doctors told me was that some men die of it and others have it and expire of something else. Anyhow, in looking around my family, I learned that I had two uncles who also had prostate cancer and they expired. And I had six first cousins who had it. Then my youngest brother developed it shortly after me. He had a radical prostatectomy but expired within two years. I believe his death was the result of the cancer going throughout his body. I had another younger brother who got it and survived. He had treatment that consisted of the use of seeds. Knowing all this, I encouraged my sons to get the PSA test at that time; the youngest one was thirty-six and he was in the military. He had an elevated PSA—it was 2. A year later, it jumped to 4—two whole points! He went and got a biopsy, and it showed he had prostate cancer. He decided that he would have it out."

Lloyd's wife, Geneva, was at home when he came in and quietly told her that he had prostate cancer. "I was distraught," she recalled. "Lloyd got very depressed. My first concern was, how bad is it? Had it metastasized? And what was life going to be like now? We had three children. What was going to happen to us? All kinds of things were going through my head. He couldn't accept it at first. I was working in the school system then, and I remember that we didn't hear much about prostate cancer. You heard a lot about breast cancer, but you didn't hear much about prostate cancer. Cancer as it relates to African American men just wasn't talked about. I tried to be supportive. Get him to open up. That was hard. I found initially he had a lot of trouble communicating with me how he was feeling."

Lloyd told Geneva he had been given two options. One was the radical prostatectomy and the second was radiation. He explained why he thought surgery was probably the way to go. "The doctor said if you have the radiation first, then you can't have the surgery afterwards. But if you have the surgery first, you *can* have radiation—if the cancer comes back." Geneva says he wanted to go through all kinds of alternatives, then talked about surgery. But he kept putting off his decision. Time passed, and Lloyd found his PSA had jumped to 70 and he had to make a choice. Geneva says he fixated on the sexual aspects of the treatments. "I urged him to get a prostatectomy. I told him I was more concerned about his living than about the sexuality. He finally accepted my suggestion."

Said Lloyd, "A week before my scheduled surgery, I got a call from a lady I had worked with back when I was at NASA. We hadn't spoken for nearly three years and she was wondering how I was doing. I told her that the following week I would be going in for surgery. And she prayed for me over the telephone. This woman has been a very religious person, with many members of her family being of the cloth. She invited me to come to the family church where her brother was the minister. And the whole church prayed for me. Then two or three days before the surgery, another woman called me. She and I had been in a play together, and she said she was calling to seek employment opportunities for her son who had just come out of the navy. And when I told her that I was undergoing surgery within two days, she prayed for me. And then she called on one of her colleagues at work who she maintained was an intercessor, and this person prayed over the telephone for me and said I would be all right. All three of them said that. And armed with that, and the fact that the church, too, had prayed for me, I went and told the doctor that the surgery is now off! He was quite disturbed, and I left.

"The following day the doctor called me and said he had three friends, all pathologists, who looked at my slides, and their conclusion was that my cancer was a fast-growing and ugly cancer and that I needed to have my prostate removed. So I reluctantly consented. But then I asked him if he would do a frozen section—which means he would take a snippet from the lymph node tissue next to the prostate and send it off to the lab to see if it was cancerous. And if it wasn't cancerous, he would get out of there and sew me back up. He reluctantly agreed to do that. I had my surgery at the University of Maryland on March 4, 1993. When I woke up, I realized the prostatectomy had been performed. And the doctor told me he saw where the prayers had benefited me inasmuch as during the surgery the prostate seemed to have lifted right up into his hands. And I thought that was wonderful! And I needed to spread the word about my plight and what was discovered, and my life was saved—based on the PSA test. I wanted to talk about all that with black men inasmuch as prostate cancer is not new to black men and they have been and still are so reluctant to see doctors. I'm committed to telling them that you can survive prostate cancer."

Lloyd's urologist was convinced his operation had been a complete success. Soon after the surgery, his PSA dropped to zero. "I insisted on having these PSA tests on a regular basis. I would have had them done every month if the health benefits people would have approved it. But they would only go for quarterly PSAs. In November of 1994, fourteen months after my prostatectomy, my PSA started creeping up again. And when my urologist called to tell me that the cancer had come back, I was floored. After my surgery I had been going around giving talks, telling men and women about the PSA test, when I learned the cancer had come back, I was naturally quite disturbed. I asked my doctor what my options were, and he told me the next thing would be to do external beam radiation. I would have to have radiation for five weeks. I was so shocked that I started experiencing problems sleeping. Even with medications . . . stronger and stronger medications. And still they didn't help. I stopped making rounds telling people how good the PSA test was and I became withdrawn and went into deep depression. The urologist suggested that I go for counseling, and I did. Indeed, I met a counselor for six long years! And finally—finally, that counselor was able to get me over my fears, and I had many.

"Meantime, I had gone back to the University of Maryland for the radiation treatments. My PSA went down to zero again and I felt so good about that. Yet I couldn't fully trust that the cancer was gone. But when I began feeling better with counseling, I started again to encourage a lot of other men to undergo counseling too, if they felt a need, as I did. The radiation was causing me to have incontinence again, and that became another problem to deal with." Geneva said, "I don't know what kept *me* going. I guess it was our religion. I prayed. We both prayed."

Lloyd continued having PSA tests done. "In 2001 I went to the VA hospital for a check-up and was told by a physician there that the cancer had come back a second time!" Lloyd rejected any suggestion that he undergo chemotherapy this time. "My youngest brother had endured a great deal of suffering as the result of chemotherapy after his prostatectomy. He became terribly disfigured and dropped from a robust one hundred and seventy pounds down to eighty-two pounds and then expired." He had heard about great successes at Johns Hopkins and decided to put himself in the hands of doctors there.

Doctors at Hopkins began a series of collagen injections spread over several months, but the procedures failed to stem the urinary flow. Their next step was to implant an artificial sphincter. It worked for a time, but later Lloyd was once more having leakage. That's when Lloyd took his incontinence issue to the nearby

VA hospital, where doctors installed a cuff around the artificial sphincter. Not long after, a second cuff was needed. At the same time, VA physicians, in a seemingly heroic procedure, injected Botox on three occasions and added the medication Vesicare to decrease Lloyd's sense of urinary urgency. His case is regarded by physicians who treated him as one of the more difficult prostate cancer issues to resolve. His PSA, with some occasional spikes, has remained at around 1.

Lloyd Bowser's traumatic experience with prostate cancer reignited his mission to save African American men. He continues to preach his gospel of salvation from this scourge. You can save yourself from cancer, he tells black men. You can be a victim or you can be a survivor. It is all up to you! "When I went to Hopkins, I helped formulate their support group, called the Man to Man program, and what we're telling men who have been diagnosed and who are about to undergo a cancer procedure is how to deal with prostate problems. We offer encouragement and support. For a variety of reasons, many African American men don't trust doctors and hospitals. This distrust of doctors and hospitals has caused many black men to avoid seeing doctors, at their own peril. When I talk to black men, what I have to offer them is a message of hope. There's hope in the fact that I have survived now for sixteen years. There is so much out there now that can help men. When I got the cancer, there were no support groups that I was aware of. I was just left in total confusion. All that has changed now. The hope that I would leave to men today—black and all—is that our doctors are moving ahead through research. Plus, there is so much hope now that you're no longer going to be butchered by somebody who doesn't have the technical skills, the knowledge skills, and the ability to handle the problems that men manifest when they have prostate cancer.

"Today, I am really upbeat! I am alive! And I thought at one time I wouldn't get to see any grandchildren. I didn't get any grandchildren until 2002. But I do now, and I have lived to be able to spend time with them. I'm a survivor of prostate cancer now for fourteen years." Adds Geneva, "I think we have a better relationship now than we ever had because we both learned to communicate more, to understand that life is tenuous, and we have learned to be more open and more loving."

For whatever reason, when prostate cancer invaded Lloyd's body, surgical intervention failed him. The probability is that his prostatectomy left behind some microscopic cancer cells that migrated throughout his body, where they grew and caused two recurrences. Radiation to destroy those cells did not locate all of them, and over time the errant cells blossomed into a second recurrence. Repeat radiation would have exposed him to complications and was not possible. He has chosen a course of expectant management for now, hoping his condition remains stable and under control. It is clear that had Lloyd Bowser's cancer been detected earlier, his initial outcome might have been more successful.

The Doctor's Notebook

Lloyd Bowser and his wife offer a message of hope. They tell of his very difficult ordeal with prostate cancer. His condition represents perhaps one of the more serious presentations of prostate cancer in terms of the threat of the disease. He experienced a delayed diagnosis and subsequently delayed treatment. There were two recurrences, and at the time of his interview, while his cancer remained under control, it was apparently persisting. He continued with a surveillance mode, understanding that his disease was not fully cured. Adding to this weight of the problem, Lloyd had a very strong family history of prostate cancer. It is sad that his younger brother had succumbed to the disease. His younger brother had both an aggressive head and neck cancer and prostate cancer. He underwent a successful radical prostatectomy, but he died of his other cancer. All in all, it is no wonder Lloyd experienced deep depression surrounding this disease.

Despite his harsh reality, Lloyd proclaims a strong message that you can survive prostate cancer. Clearly, disease eradication is the ultimate goal once the diagnosis is made. This goal may be difficult to achieve, however, if the cancer has progressed at the time of diagnosis. Lloyd and his wife observe that they initially interpreted the disease as having consequences on his sexuality and sexual function. They learned subsequently that this and other adverse effects of the disease and his treatment are actually minor concerns. Fortunately, with better treatments offered today, the side effects are also minimized. Nonetheless, particular emphasis should be given to the importance of life. As it has been said, without life there is no quality of life.

Without question, Lloyd is a proponent of proactive management of the disease. I salute him for initiating a support group for men with prostate cancer. As he recognizes, more are needed. In this belief he echoes the purpose of this book.

21

Gabe Daniels

No Love Lost: "Just Between Us Boys . . ."

Gabe Daniels is not his real name. Because of the frankness expressed in this interview, we have agreed to withhold his true identity. Except for information that might reveal his identity, the facts stated here are true and his remarks are faithful and accurate to the best of his recollections.

Gabe Daniels runs a family-owned service business and lives in New York City with his significant other, who works in broadcasting. Both were sixty at the time of this interview in January 2008. For the purpose of this story, we refer to Gabe's partner as Valerie.

Gabe and Valerie first met in the seventh grade and by sheer chance were reunited years later after his happy marriage of twenty-four years ended when his wife suddenly died. The couple's only son had tragically died in infancy. When Valerie and Gabe met again, he was still single. She had been divorced, and the two decided to live together. Today, both of Valerie's daughters are grown. Gabe and Valerie are still together after fifteen years.

Gabe is a tall, heavyset man with salt-and-pepper hair. He wears silver-rimmed glasses, and his dress is as casual as his manner. He's pleasant and full of good humor and comfortable to be around. Above all, he is a very private man who, while guarding his true identity, is not afraid to express his thoughts and feelings with great candor. Why? Because he wants people to know what it's like to have prostate cancer and learn to deal with it. Cancer is not new to Daniels. "A number of people in my family had cancer. My father died of Hodgkin's disease [cancer of the lymphatic system, which is part of the immune system]. My mother had breast cancer twice! My sister died of ovarian cancer. Both of my grandfathers probably had prostate cancer, but we don't know for sure. We just think so."

Gabe always tried to make sure he was in good health. "I always do treadmill walking in the morning, and living in the city requires that you walk a lot, which is a good thing. And I've always been in some sports. I'm an avid golfer. I play quite a bit of golf in the summertime. I'm also a fisherman. I started as a kid, down at the Jersey shore. My grandfather had a place down there. Today, I have a small boat and do a lot of fishing, mostly in Long Island Sound. So I try to keep in shape."

His introduction to his prostate began when he was in his middle to late forties. "I started having urinary problems, and I went to the doctor and he did a digital exam. He determined that I had an enlarged prostate. A few years after, the urinary problems were such that I felt I needed medication, and I was sent to a urologist. That helped, and then I went to him for the next few years and he began giving me PSA tests. The numbers, he said, were okay, but they were on the high side of okay.

"In the late nineties, the urologist decided to do a biopsy and found no particular problems. We waited another year or two and did biopsies again. Then—I think it was in the early part of 2001—he told me I had prostate cancer in a couple of the core samples. I was fifty-four when I was diagnosed. The thing is that all along the PSAs were showing the high end of normal. Up to that point, all he had been saying is that he didn't find anything abnormal, just that the prostate had become enlarged. The medication he'd given me did help with my urinating problem. I was going less frequently but doing more urinating [stronger stream] each time, rather than going more often and not as having as much urine each time.

"When the urologist told me I had prostate cancer, I was . . . well, I would have to say, stunned. I told myself, 'I'm gonna die! I'm gonna die!' He sat down and told me what his findings were. And he also discussed what my possible options were. Surgery . . . and seeds . . . and radiation . . . and combinations thereof. Or not doing anything. He was a surgeon, but he suggested that I check out the other options—that is, consult with people who do those other methods. I went and saw a second urologist, someone who did seeds and radiation. And he explained to me how they do seeds and how they work. I didn't speak with anyone who actually had the seeds method, but I did speak with a couple of people who had had surgery. And then I went to see yet another urologist that did surgery. And on his recommendation, my conclusion was that as long as the prostate was in there—whether I had seeds or radiation or not—that I could still have a recurrence.

"I was in therapy at the time—psychoanalysis. I wasn't there for sexual reasons necessarily, but it's all part of my life, so I decided to bring the subject up. I decided to talk about it. Talking to the therapist helped. But what I think helped more was talking with Valerie. She was my biggest support for it all. The support on her side was, 'Yeah, it's awful. Yeah, it's terrible. But the information out there is that you don't have to die from it . . . if you do surgery—and that's what we're being told.' Now, the seeds and radiation work for people, too. The thing that bothered me more than anything, though—and I may be wrong about this— was if you did the seeds or the radiation, you can't have surgery later. That was my feeling. We, you know, we have one chance to get this devil out of there. I think Valerie was probably more anxious for me to have it out. Just so that I would be alive!"

Did Gabe and Valerie talk about the outcomes of surgery and the possibility of his losing sexual potency? "Yes, I was upset about it, and I'm sure she was upset about it. Her feeling was she didn't want me to die, we would work that out somehow. I decided on surgery and had it done at the New York University Medical Center. I think the whole idea here was survival. Our feeling was and is that there's more to sex than intercourse, and [more to] a loving partner than intercourse. And frankly, at the time, the information I was being given was that intercourse was probably going to be in an eighty to ninety percent range, and that things would return to normal."

And just how did things work out for Gabe? "The incontinence part of it in the beginning was very weird. Obviously, you wear pads or diapers all the time. I did that for six months! It was annoying. It was troublesome. I got used to it. In the beginning, you changed very often and you'd be very wet. Later on, you wouldn't change so often and you weren't nearly as wet. You know, nobody wants to walk around with wet pants. It's not fun. It took a lot of planning, and the only time I nearly panicked was on 9/11. I was on a plane to California on my way for a golf vacation, and then it all happened. We landed in Ohio, and they shuttled us off to a hotel, but we couldn't get our baggage. It had been checked in and I only had a couple of pads in a little carry-on bag. And I had no means to get any more. I eventually found out there was a mall down the road, and I walked down there and found a drugstore; then I was home free. But, ya know, for the whole time I'm sitting on the plane in Ohio I was alone, and that was quite troublesome . . . wondering, what the heck was I gonna do? But that worked out.

"Now, [as for] the outcome of the sexual thing. It was my understanding that I had a seventy-five to eighty percent chance of having erections afterward. I had the nerve-sparing thing. So, you know, I was playing the numbers. Okay, I don't want to have the cancer . . . I don't want to be wet. Okay, we can probably deal with that, and I'd like to have an erection now and then. One, two, three—that was about the right priority. As it turned out, it's now seven years and I haven't had an erection without the use of injections!"

What was that like? Does it work for Gabe? "Well, the answer is yes *and* no. Yes, it works. Let me explain. First of all, the first time I injected myself, I'm sitting there thinking, 'What the *hell* am I doing? Sticking a needle in my penis! My God! You gotta be kidding.' So I go ahead and do it. And yeah, it burns because you have a drug in it. It becomes hard and a little bit . . . uh . . . uncomfortable. And I don't know if it's from the surgery or what, but my penis now breaks hard to the left or right. I can't remember now which way, but it's got a little hook to it and it's shorter than

I remember! I was never told that would happen. I do know now. I do know that it's because when they reconnect you they have to pull it in a little bit. Well, nobody told me that. And I've never been the one with the ten-inch penis to start with . . . I didn't have much to waste! To complete this little discussion, I wanna add this about the injection. It not only burns, but it feels very strange. The penis hooks to the left or right, as I said, and I want to describe the sensation. It's as though you just slammed it in a car door. It's sort of . . . *oooh*! And then obviously you can have penetration at that point. Of course, your mind is on your penis. It's not on your partner at that point. So it's not about all the other lovemaking things. You're thinking about your penis. Well, you might as well be with yourself then. And also there's no ejaculate. There isn't the same feeling. You don't have that same sort of climax that you would normally have."

What reaction does Valerie have to Gabe's injection-induced erection? Does the partner have a different experience? Gabe says, "We didn't use it enough to . . . well, it was like, 'Oh, God, we did it!' It was like a chore. And okay, we did it this time, but okay we did that . . . and then we haven't done that in a long time. It was so uncomfortable, and very honestly, we haven't had any penetration in probably five years.

"And yet the two of us have survived. You know, there are other things you can do to please her, and that's fine. But honestly I don't feel like I have the same desire that I had, and it hasn't anything to do with her. I love her to death. I think she's beautiful. I don't have the same libido that I used to have, and I don't know if that's part of being sixty or whether it's part of the surgery. Or whether it's part of this blocking the whole idea of the thing. Valerie is a terrific partner, but sometimes she'll say to me, 'It's almost like I'm living with my brother.' We don't have as much intimacy as we would like to have.

"Let me say something that I think is the most important to bring out. The incontinence part cleared up after a certain amount of time . . . the difficulties that maybe Valerie and I still deal with as far as having sex with each other. Remember, the number one reason I had the surgery was that I would live and wouldn't have cancer. And that's the most important part of this whole thing. What people need to remember is that if you don't live, it doesn't matter whether you can have an erection or not. Because you're not having an erection if you're dead!

"So, getting rid of the prostate cancer is the most important part. You can survive. You can do other things, and I have work to do. In those last couple of years, Valerie and I have said we have to try to do something about our sexuality and stuff. It isn't that she's gonna leave me or that I'm gonna leave her. You gotta work on it. And I think that's probably true of all people, even people that don't have prostate cancer surgery. Whether it's marriage or people living together, we all have to work at it. It's a people thing. I have heard that penile implants work a lot better, without all the troubles I talked about. And I am thinking about it, maybe down the road. The fact that you think you're never gonna have sex the way you remember it again—yeah, that's pretty tough. It's not easy, you know. It's part of life. I've had a lot of problems in my life, but I also know there are always good things in my life. And that's why I try to look forward to the good things. You know, I had a wife for twenty-four years and she died. And a few years later, I'm with Valerie. I've had two women that love me. Most guys have trouble finding one. I'm pretty lucky." Somewhere in there, Gabe Daniels told us, there's a lesson for everybody.

The Doctor's Notebook

Gabe Daniels seems to be a fine fellow whom we all would like to meet. He has such a mild-mannered way of being and a definite humorous side, and he has such a great perspective on life. His narrative of his personal experience with receiving a diagnosis of prostate cancer and then taking action to rid himself of this disease is funny yet compelling. In a lot of respects, the story is familiar to many. Those men who receive regular medical check-ups may find that increasing attention is given to their prostate health. I salute Gabe and others for continuing with such a diligent health-care program. In his case, because of the concern of a rising PSA measurement and a family history of prostate cancer, he received careful medical evaluations that eventually confirmed his diagnosis. He seemed to handle the entire experience of treatment and recovery in a noble way.

Gabe discusses a major health issue associated with any prostate cancer treatment, including surgery: altered sexual function. It seems that he endured setbacks in a host of areas relating to the male sexual response. Despite a nerve-sparing approach to radical prostatectomy, which is intended to maximize sexual function recovery, he did not recover his erectile function. Besides experiencing erectile dysfunction, he also observed a penile deformity, orgasmic changes, and a lowering of his libido. All of these conditions can indeed occur in a man who has undergone radical prostatectomy. Let me take this opportunity to review the matter of sexual changes after radical prostatectomy.

Erectile dysfunction can occur in many men after radical prostatectomy, despite the innovation of the anatomic nerve-sparing technique approximately twenty-five years ago. In the era prior to this innovation, erectile dysfunction following the surgery was universal. A better understanding of the requirements for penile erection included definition of the nerves responsible for regulating penile erection that course through the pelvis and terminate in the penis. After the description of the surgery by Dr. Patrick C. Walsh in a more anatomic approach, nerve preservation was improved and many men were able to recover erections.

However, even with meticulous surgical technique, the nerves for erection in the pelvis can be traumatized during surgery to the extent that all men experience some level of erectile dysfunction at first. As the nerves regain function, many men will eventually recover erectile function. At the same time, many will not, for unclear reasons. Many factors influence the eventuality of erectile dysfunction following radical prostatectomy. These include nerve and blood vessel trauma at the time of surgery; other adverse health conditions, ranging from age to cardiovascular disease; and relationship difficulties that many men may experience in the course of their lives at this time. It is important to recognize these factors, despite the best attempts by the surgeon to preserve structures critical for the erection response.

Penile deformity has also been observed in men undergoing radical prostatectomy. This ranges from obvious scar tissue development within the penis, with angulation, to minor changes of tissue damage within the penis that may not be so readily observed by physical examination. These changes can affect the mechanical properties of blood flow associated with penile erection, or can alter the position of the penis in sexual intercourse. The scientific basis for these changes remain unclear at this time. Some investigators in this field have postulated that the lack of circulation to the penis in the postoperative course of several months affects the health of erectile tissue such that it becomes deformed. Fortunately, this does not occur in the majority of men.

Orgasmic function changes are common following radical prostatectomy, to the extent that a true ejaculate is not possible after the prostate and seminal vesicles have been removed. In my professional experience, many men have expressed to me that they preserve the sensation of orgasm although fluid emission is absent. Some men may have heightened orgasmic experiences following the surgery, whereas others encounter uncomfortable or even painful experiences. For the latter, much of this can be addressed medically, or the noxious sensations may abate over time.

Changes in a man's libido may occur following radical prostatectomy or indeed any treatment for prostate cancer. Some of this may relate to the reduction in the overall sexual experience that then secondarily reduces a man's interest in pursuing sexual activity. If the sexual experience is less dramatically affected, many men will preserve their libido.

Gabe tells of how he confronted his sexual dysfunction. Clearly, an element of his recovery was that he had a loving partner, and the importance of this should not be underestimated. He also jocularly stated the truism that erections are not possible if you are not alive. This statement reflects the perspective that all matters of one's life can be handled, including sexual problems, as long as the prostate cancer has been cured and one is alive to pursue management options. Indeed, Gabe took a positive approach to his management options, electing to move forward with penile injection therapy to achieve erections. Again, I applaud him for his forthrightness and initiative.

Let me take this moment to provide a doctor's discussion about the penile injection treatment option. In the management of erectile dysfunction, including that following radical prostatectomy, penile injection therapy represents a second-line option, with the first-line option being oral medications such as Viagra, Levitra, and Cialis. In men who do not respond to oral treatment, second-line management in the form of penile injection therapy can be considered. This is a pharmacologic approach in which medication that mimics natural chemicals that induce an erection is delivered by direct injection into the penis. Men can be taught how to perform the technique of self-injection, in a dose sufficient to produce an erection that lasts approximately thirty minutes. It is important that the erection last only a sufficient time to be useful for sexual intercourse. The medication standardly used initially is prostaglandin E1, also known as alprostadil, which causes some transient achy sensation in the penis that Gabe referred to. Only a small proportion of men experience the sensation, and over time many find it to be less uncomfortable. Indeed, the medication is safe to use and is preferred as the vasoactive drug of choice for this purpose. Other medications can be used, such as papaverine and phentolamine, but these may yield a more unpredictable response in producing an erection and more frequently cause erectile tissue scar formation. This form of therapy should be offered only under the supervision of a urologist who is familiar with how these medications are used and can respond if a complication occurs. If this treatment is less desirable, the alternative second-line treatment of vacuum erection device therapy can be applied. In some men for whom penile injection therapy does not work, is contraindicated, or seems unsatisfactory, the third-line option of penile prosthesis surgery can be explored.

22

Robert Piscotty and Mary Anne Piscotty

Climbing a Steep Mountain of Medical Complexities One Step at a Time

Robert Piscotty, a retired Pennsylvania state policeman, lives in the rural town of York Springs, not far from Harrisburg, the state capital. He built the house with his own hands and assistance from one of his two sons. It is a lovely single-story dwelling with a finished basement and lots of storage. His wife, Mary Anne, a bubbly and expressive brunette, tends to the large garden surrounding their home. She is frequently found baking or cooking in their spacious kitchen. The Piscottys have four grown children, two boys and two girls. To describe them as simply a warm couple would be an understatement. They are exceedingly hospitable to all who enter their home. Hugs are almost guaranteed.

Robert is a large man with a beaming smile and a great sense of humor. At the time of this interview in March 2008, he was about to turn sixty-nine, which he said he could not believe. He prefers that his friends call him Bob. He grew up in Plymouth, a small town just outside of Wilkes-Barre, Pennsylvania. His father was a coal miner who lived to be eighty, and he told Bob that if he ever considered following his footsteps into the mine he would break his legs. He suggested that Bob consider becoming a state trooper, and in 1960, when he was twenty-one, that is precisely what Bob Piscotty decided to do. He stayed on the job until 1990, when he made up his mind to retire. For Bob, retirement did not mean becoming a couch potato. He is a man with an itch to be active, and as he will tell you, he "always has to be into something." That "something" was often building and repairing houses for his children, friends, and himself and his wife. He has tried to stay active in sports, too, and when he was employed, he organized a state police softball team and a basketball team. These days you may find Bob running or fooling around with the old 1948 Ford tractor that he uses to keep the grounds in good shape. There are few mechanical things that Bob Piscotty cannot handle—except maybe a computer! That is, of course, a digital device, and Bob is content being an analog man.

For a long time he had been getting physicals only sporadically. But when he turned fifty, he knew it was time to start seeing a doctor more regularly. "Back then I was helping build my boy's home that he's living in right now. It was about that time I started having physicals. That's when I discovered I had a problem with my heart. They told me my heart rhythm was off. I was really overweight, too. I was pushing two hundred eighty pounds. Nowadays I get my physicals at the Veterans Administration, and I do that every year." Things for Bob Piscotty were on a roll until around 2002. "I had an ablation in 2002 [a medical procedure utilizing electric stimulation to control arrhythmia or irregular heartbeats]. It worked out fine for a while, but then sometime in 2006 I started feeling bad."

Mary Anne picks up the story. "In June, he started feeling poorly, his heart went into afib [atrial fibrillation, an irregular and often rapid heart rate that commonly causes poor blood flow to the body; symptoms are heart palpitations, shortness of breath, and weakness]. He goes down to Johns Hopkins in Baltimore to see a cardiologist about a second ablation. He was scheduled to have this done in September of 2006. Before they could proceed, they had to do a CT scan of his chest and they found spots on his lungs. At that point, the doctor says they couldn't do the ablation. He sent Bob home to have his lung problem checked out. It took a month and a half to get an appointment at Hershey Hospital. The doctors at Hershey Hospital did an endoscopy and a biopsy of the lung and ruled out TB [tuberculosis] and cancer. They then approved an ablation for Bob and scheduled it for February 2007. Long before February rolled around, Bob couldn't even walk up a flight of stairs. He'd come in from the driveway and have to sit down in a chair and more or less collapse and gasp for air. We just said, 'We're headed back to Hopkins!' Bob's Hopkins cardiologist was still unable to do the ablation. By now the oxygen level in his blood was only 86 and it needed to be at least at 93 before they would even attempt an operation. They pulled in a pulmonary team to get to the bottom of his lung problem. They took all kinds of tests, including a lung biopsy. They came back with a diagnosis of rheumatoid arthritis of the lungs, something they said was a very rare condition. He was also suffering from interstitial pneumonia [inflammation of the lung tissues]. They put him on medications for pulmonary therapy and we went home and took things one day at a time. Finally he began to feel better."

It was now the end of December 2006, time for Bob to have his annual physical check-up. His primary physician in Hershey called to tell him his PSA was high. "My PSA had been between 1 and 2 for the longest time. And all of a sudden it went to 4.2. That jump was over three years, and my doctor said I should get it checked out by a urologist, and she recommended one. I was having no symptoms . . . nothing, no indications whatsoever. This urologist in Harrisburg gave me the DRE. And afterwards he did an endoscopy and biopsies. Then he sat me down and came right out with it. He said, 'You have cancer of the prostate, and it has to be taken care of.' He told me the PSA was a little over 4, but he never gave me a Gleason [score]. I just sat there and listened to the options. He said, 'Yours is an extremely slow-moving cancer . . . not aggressive.' He said, 'You can do expectant management and you can live ten years, maybe twenty; you don't know.' It didn't shake me up, though, and that's when he said, 'You can have the prostate removed or we can treat it with radiation.' I said, 'Well, I'll think about it,' and he gave me the literature. He said, 'I can make an appointment with a surgeon in Hershey at a local hospital if you want,' and told me to make up my mind which way I wanted to go."

Mary Anne was not with him at the time. "I only found out about it when he came home from the doctor's," she says. "I was very shocked. With everything else that was going on, I was scared for him. I knew things were happening in his body and I saw how quickly he was going downhill—from June seemingly when nothing was wrong with him to now when was having all these things bombarding him at once! I tried to encourage him to go see the best doctor he could. And he told me he didn't feel good about the doctors in Harrisburg. He said the one he saw told him he could do watchful waiting, but he never gave Bob the Gleason number. We talked about it and both decided he should go back to Hopkins. He had a cardiologist there, and we thought he would be a good person to help him find a doctor to give him a second opinion. Actually, when the urologist in Harrisburg told Bob he could hold off and just do expectant management, I felt a little more secure in the sense that we could wait a little while. But then Bob suddenly made his decision right there and then."

Bob says he decided that the thing for him to do was to have surgery. "I based my decision on some chats I had with some guys I like to hang out with. There I was shooting the breeze with them. One guy—a poker buddy of mine—I didn't know he had prostate cancer until I started telling him about mine. And he said, yeah, he had had prostate cancer and he got it removed. He says he went up to a hospital in Pennsylvania and had it done and he's doing okay. Then he tells me he could have had seeds or radiation, but he had the operation and it worked out."

Once Bob's mind was made up, Mary Anne went about gathering research material. "I got hold of the Dr. Patrick Walsh book [*Dr. Patrick Walsh's Guide to Surviving Prostate Cancer*] on how to deal with prostate cancer and I read some parts of it. But we were all caught up with his lung problem and doing everything step by step every day, you know. We were going a day at a time, not knowing what the next day would bring. And when he started bouncing back [as a result of the prescribed lung medications], well, then we started zeroing in on what to do about his prostate. And we drove down to Baltimore and saw Dr. Galindez, a urologist down there. Dr. Galindez wanted to know how come Bob waited so long to see him. That's when he told us that Bob had a

Gleason score of 7! Dr. Galindez told us that the surgery option was out—off the table—because his lungs and his heart weren't in any kind of shape to undergo an operation and they were afraid to put him under anesthesia."

Says Bob, "The way Dr. Galindez put it to me was, 'Bob, there's no way you will find a doctor here at Johns Hopkins that will do surgery on you to remove your prostate.' And then he sent me down to confer with his colleague, Dr. Chan Lee, to see if he would suggest seeds or external radiation. I sat down with Dr. Lee—my wife and I—and he said he thought seeds would be best for me, but first he had to make sure I was a candidate for seed implants. So he says we're gonna find out. And he scheduled some tests. They went up my rectum and tested the prostate to see if I was eligible and concluded I was. I don't think Mary Anne or I were frightened. I feel that what I done is the right course, and I feel good right now. My wife, whatever decision I made, she was very supportive."

Mary Anne was completely stressed out. "When I looked at him and saw how he was failing back in February and how he was struggling to get through it, I admired him for his inner strength . . . and if this seed implant was the thing to help him . . . I wanted it to be the right thing for him. Actually, I didn't talk to too many people about what was going on. I will say I prayed a lot. I didn't have much time really to dwell on it, but each night when you say your prayers, you pray to the Big Guy. Let the Lord help. He's there for you. He certainly was there for us."

Bob had trouble recalling much about his brachytherapy treatment because he feel asleep almost immediately after the procedure began. "I think they said they put in sixty-seven seeds. When I awoke it was eight o'clock at night. I either had to go home or I could have stayed in a room down there. I had to be back the next morning. I told them I'd go home because I was only two hours away. I had the catheter in me, early the next morning my wife drove me back down—catheter and all—I went in there, and to my relief they removed the catheter. They wouldn't let me go home again until I could to the bathroom on my own. Then Dr. Lee said, 'So long. See you in May for further tests.'

"After my procedure, I was running to the bathroom for a little bit and they gave me some pills to take care of it. That worked and I haven't had any urinary problems since then. One thing Dr. Lee did tell me was not to have sexual relations for ninety days. It's possible seeds may come out during ejaculation. I also had to chuckle to myself because I had been suffering from ED and I couldn't have sexual relations if I wanted to. He also told me I was not to have any children sit on my lap, try not to get too close to anybody for any length of time, because you don't want anybody to be exposed to radiation. I had the seed procedure in September, so tomorrow it will be nine months."

Over time, Bob began feeling so well that his thoughts returned to his problem of ED. He had tried Cialis and Viagra in the past, but neither worked for him. He considered trying a vacuum pump and injections but rejected both. Ultimately, he called Johns Hopkins for help. They put him in touch with Dr. Burnett. He and Dr. Burnett had quite a talk, and that's when he learned about a penile implant. Bob is quite an authority on penile implants now. "It's more or less a pump. They insert two tubes in the penis and there's a reservoir of fluids with the pump. You squeeze it and pump up your penis to whatever size you want for however long you want. It's about the size of a marble. It's not visible and nobody can tell. I had it inserted a little over a month ago. Using the implant, I found, is not embarrassing at all, not whatsoever. My wife and I talked about it and I had to wait for the incision to heal. It's been over a month now. And I was really looking forward to trying it out. It doesn't bother you when you walk around. When you use it in the beginning, it was a little sore, but I was told it would get better when I fully healed. And it's already getting better. I tried it just today and it works great. I experimented using the pump at the doctor's office—he showed me how it works. Then when I came home I experimented with it, and in bed this morning it worked great. If you ask how long the erection lasts, well, that's really up to you. If you pump it up, the only way it's gonna go down is there's a release inside—inside your scrotum. You just press the release—so you really control the length of time."

Bob anticipates that once he masters the penile implant he will be one happy man. "I think it will be the greatest thing that's happened." Does Bob believe his wife can tell the difference between a natural erection and a penile implant? "No. Like I said, we haven't had much time with it yet. It's something new and something to work at."

"I'll tell you what," Mary Anne says, laughing. "Bob had his chance last night. And this was a day or two after he saw his doctor. He came home and I asked him how it had gone. He said fine, but he was a little sore still, and I told him it was understandable. I don't pressure him. I said, 'When you're ready, you'll tell me.' So, actually last night he said he was ready. And it was funny because we use this special little word . . . poor little Willie. Will he *will* or Willie Wonka? So, it was one of those things, you know. We found out about wee Willie and Willie Wonka last night. Actually, he was . . . how can I say it? When you're getting used to a new toy, this is what I made the comparison to. It's just a new little toy. We're gonna learn how to work with it. And we're just gonna have a new little life because being little virgins like we are now . . . we're gonna have to work through it. To me, it's a little different, okay? But I think it'll get better because I don't really think that he's learned how to work it properly, you know. And he wants me to work it properly. And this is what I told him, and, of course, he asked me. It was fine, you know, but it's like getting married again. You have to work all the little things. Like you're trying to find all the little buttons. Is this the right button? What does it feel like? Where do you have your hand? Where should I put my hand? And so, you learn the proper ways to do it, you know. I think it'll be a fabulous thing! I really do! And for him, I think it was the greatest thing. It *is* the greatest thing."

The Doctor's Notebook

Bob Piscotty tells about how he regained an important aspect of his life, the ability to engage in sexual intercourse with his wife. His erectile dysfunction had become complete after undergoing radiation therapy for his prostate cancer. He had successfully undergone radiation therapy and was ready to resume life. However, he clearly was not content with having erectile dysfunction. He had initially been proactive about the problem and become informed about treatment options. As with many men, first-line treatment (oral medication) and second-line treatment (vacuum erection device therapy, penile injection therapy) either did not work or were unappealing. He eventually took the third-line option, which was penile prosthesis surgery. He has shared with me that this has significantly added to his quality of life.

The penile prosthesis device can be used proficiently once a man is instructed in how to use it. It does not interfere with other aspects of life, and it is convenient for spontaneous sexual intercourse. Indeed, Bob fully understood his wife's message that love is more important than sex. But as his case demonstrates, it is possible to have sexual ability in addition to a loving relationship. The message is clear to me that men do not have to accept loss of sexual activity for the rest of their lives just because they underwent prostate cancer treatment in any form, including radiation therapy. Options exist to manage erectile dysfunction resulting from prostate cancer treatment. The key is to have a frank conversation with a specialist in sexual medicine who can present the alternatives in a balanced and supportive way and then help the patient decide what is the best intervention. Penile prosthesis surgery may seem a daunting ordeal for many, but as Bob's case shows, it can be done quite acceptably with highly satisfactory results.

The Future

Treatments and Perspectives

Once the world of prostate cancer was a world of despair. Today, that world is one of hope. Once men with the disease often faced death or a life of pain and misery. Today, men who are diagnosed early survive and continue leading life to the fullest. Thanks to the rapidity of scientific and medical advances, even men with the most challenging prostate cases can look forward to new procedures and treatments to help prolong their lives and renew their hopes.

The first major development came in 1982 when Dr. Patrick C. Walsh, then professor and director of the Brady Urological Institute at the Johns Hopkins Hospital, performed the first nerve-sparing operation during a radical open prostatectomy. For skilled surgeons everywhere it became a mountain-moving surgical procedure, drastically reducing the risks of urinary incontinence and erectile dysfunction. In the late 1980s, the PSA as a screening tool came into wider acceptance. For men with advanced prostate cancer, however, treatments were slower in coming; for them, it was a course of steady decline with little help even from chemotherapy. All of that is changing. Oncologists today have found the means of predicting those at risk of cancer recurrence, and researchers are hard at work testing new drugs and therapies to deal with advanced cancer and carrying out clinical trials.

Despite all of the progress and all of the advances that have been made so far against prostate cancer, we cannot in all honesty conclude that we have won the war. How far have we come and how far must we go? For an assessment, we turn to Dr. Burnett.

Where do you believe we need improvements in dealing with prostate cancer?

We need improvements in all areas of managing prostate cancer. I don't regard one more important than another. For starters, we need better early detection. There has to be more counseling to at-risk groups, letting them know that they have to get screened. We still need better education. The impact is perhaps greatest for the black community, but all men should take heed. So I would say the first place we need improvement is in awareness.

Another would be diagnosis. We need better diagnostic tools. I think our diagnostic tools at this point still are imperfect. Take, for example, biopsies. We know that men have indications to get a prostate biopsy because of an elevation in PSA, or an abnormality on prostate examination [DRE]. But from clinical experience, we find that as many as eighty percent of these patients don't have cancer! So, four or five guys then have gone through an uncomfortable procedure where we really don't find cancer. We need to do a better job trying to identify those who will need biopsy and not put guys through procedures that are tough to endure.

So there's a need in that area to improve our diagnostic tools. There are different ways that are being explored in that area. Let me give you an example.

PSA testing was introduced in the late 1980s and was a big improvement from where we were with prostate cancer management in the prior era. Before PSAs, we had to rely entirely on suspicious findings we felt on a DRE. Let's say we felt a nodule. That would prompt a prostate biopsy to confirm the diagnosis. We would then operate on these guys or take them through radiation, hoping to be effective, but knowing we were oftentimes late with our diagnosis. In truth, we were curing two out of three men. But with the introduction of the PSA test we had a much better tool to enable us to diagnose. It offered an alternative approach besides the DRE to suggest an abnormality of the prostate. So far, so good. But there is an important insight associated with the PSA test. *It is not cancer-specific.* By that I mean, *the PSA is specific for a condition of the prostate, but not for prostate cancer!* Consequently, when a man has a PSA that is abnormal [elevated], it could result from BPH [benign prostatic hyperplasia—an enlarged prostate] or from prostatitis [a noncancerous infection]. *The bottom line is that we need a better blood marker—a more precise tool that tells us of the likelihood that a man really has prostate cancer.* We need and are working on a serum biomarker that can be picked up in the bloodstream with a simple blood test that is more specific for prostate cancer proteins or antigens. One of our scientists here at Johns Hopkins, Dr. Robert Getzenberg, is currently evaluating and developing the early prostate cancer antigen test. It is called EPCA [early prostate cancer antigen]. And that test we think is likely to be a true advance if it really is confirmed.

Because the PSA test has significant limitations, more often than not a man with an elevated PSA level turns out *not* to have prostate cancer. What we are saying is that these false positive PSA results—elevated PSA levels—can lead to many unnecessary biopsies, sometimes multiple biopsies. You can readily understand the need for a better test—what we call a "test with high specificity." *One that would correctly produce a negative result when a person does not have prostate cancer!* In the meantime, urologists and researchers continue to debate what constitutes a "normal" PSA level and what is the value of an isolated PSA measurement versus how quickly a man's PSA level rises over time. While other researchers continue their work on EPCA, I would point out that additional work goes on at many other institutions as well to find better tools—new biomarkers—that will improve diagnosis and management of the disease. Ongoing investigations involve the use of blood or tissue samples subjected to evaluations such as molecular genetic studies and even nanomicrochip analysis of specific genetic matter that indicate the presence of cancer cells or reveal its aggressiveness. In sum, the amount of research under way only serves to underscore our belief that better mousetraps may be on the way.

One big problem patients often face is equivocal findings on biopsies. If the indications are not certain, the patient's decision concerning treatment becomes a true dilemma. Are we making progress on this front?

If you recall the story of Mr. Lennox Graham [chapter 16], you'll find his account is a nice example of equivocal findings. Pathologists looking under a microscope at biopsy tissue render the diagnosis that is based on visual interpretation, and that may reflect the level of training and experience of the pathologist in determining what looks like cancer under the microscope. Now, let's say we're all birdwatchers. The best birdwatchers among us do the better job. If you think about it, wouldn't you rather have faith in knowing that the pathologist at the microscope can tell for sure if what he sees are actually cancer cells? Wouldn't you rather have an accurate automated or computerized system where all the pathologists who view the slides could agree on the findings? In Mr. Graham's case, one pathologist came up with a finding of 15 percent cancerous sample, while another came up with 85 percent. One person's thought was, 'I think I'm seeing more cancer cells in this one-centimeter-long thread of tissue than the other pathologist who saw less.' The difference in opinion significantly impacted on the treatment decision. Here again is yet another instance where we have to do better.

What kinds of improvements in treatment can we look forward to?

I think we need to make improvements in this area as well. For localized prostate cancer, we made progress . . . advances in surgery . . . advances in radiation. Now there's growing interest in cryosurgery. There's interest in high-intensity focused ultrasound. We don't know what the long-term outcomes of some of these treatments are, so that's a little bit challenging. But we are moving in the direction of exploring increasingly effective therapy with less complications. That is the overall game. Is one treatment automatically superior to another? No, not in such absolute terms. Each treatment may or may not be right for the patient, depending on the circumstances of his cancer as well as the circumstances of his age and health and expectations of his longevity.

I think that brachytherapy [seed implantation] can be offered to the healthy sixty- or fifty-five-year-old guy, or even a fifty-year-old.

But clearly eligible candidates in this age bracket in my view should opt for a radical prostatectomy. However, for somebody whose limited health and longevity is a concern or maybe when there is a low-level threat of prostate cancer, surgery may not be the right thing to do. So I think every intervention has its role. In my mind, it's a matter of moving forward a little bit better—trying to determine who are the best candidates for the right therapies. It is regrettable that so far we have yet to settle open questions as to what treatment for localized disease is most effective because of the lack of controlled trials to help us figure this out. When it comes to making what could be the most important decision in their lives, about whether to have treatment or not, or what kind of treatment to have, some patients are content to work that out for themselves—doing research, gathering facts, factoring in what their doctor tells them, perhaps talking to others, and getting second opinions. Others, however, feel helpless or conflicted. They want the doctor to make the decision for them and they can get angry if the physician defers. Some doctors oblige; some don't. What is going on here?

None of us doctors are hiding anything. It's just that there are controversies in places, and we do know that patient preferences do play roles in some of the decision-making process. I think we try to be as forthright as we can where we have the information. But we also have to take a read on our patients. One will be very well informed and logical in his thinking. Others want you to do it for them. Remember the case of Mr. and Mrs. Charles Brickell [chapter 15]? Mrs. Brickell says she would be very comfortable if you just tell her what she has to do. It is not easy for the physician to make a personal decision for a patient when the course and threat of the disease is not certain.

Can you elaborate on the likely course prostate cancer treatment will take in the future?

The thrust of treatment in the future is clear: we must improve our treatment outcomes with less side effects. We've seen advances with surgery, with nerve sparing. We've seen advances in radiation in terms of IMRT [intensity-modulated radiation therapy] and more specific things like that. Still, complications arise, just because the prostate is in a very precarious part of the body. It's adjacent to the urinary control areas. It's adjacent to the nerves that are critical for erection. It's adjacent to the bowel, the rectum . . . so that's why there's been such enthusiasm for things like high-intensity focused ultrasound. The idea is that it's noninvasive and may be targeted. We must and can move forward and diagnose prostate cancer more accurately.

Consider the analogy of prostate cancer and breast cancer. With breast cancer it has become yesterday's radical mastectomy versus today's small lumpectomies. Complete removal versus partial removal. There's interest now in prostate cancer where if we develop better imaging—actually identifying where the cancer is with noninvasive imaging tools, maybe other kinds of specialized scans—we'll be able to get to target therapy, maybe external techniques can become effective. I think these things will become a reality in time. Rather than putting a man through invasive surgery, particularly if he has a low level of disease, if we can be certain that we know a cancer is seen, and be accurate. The worst thing would be to target a place where cancer is believed to be the only location, then discover it is somewhere else, because prostate cancer can be multifocal. My concept of moving forward would be: less invasive . . . external energy techniques based on good imaging . . . not having to remove the entire prostate . . . and all within the goal of effective efficacy and less side effects! Still, there is a strong caveat. If we think that [we are] coming up with new therapies that we believe are less traumatic to the body, but we are still not curing people, then shame on us. We still have to make sure we are meeting the goals of cancer control while minimizing the complications. That is the main message I have about treatment.

In our previous discussions about radical prostatectomy, we spoke about the complications of erectile dysfunction that can result following the surgery. At major centers where hundreds of these procedures are carried out every year, about 70 percent of the patients are eventually potent. Still, many men experience erectile difficulties. Radical prostatectomy is one of the most delicate and intricate operations to carry out. The issue of eliminating the complications of sexual dysfunction is one of the prime concerns of Dr. Burnett and his team of researchers. We asked him to describe the progress being made addressing the issue of complications of erectile dysfunction following surgery.

What we are asking here is, can't we do better with the realities of the treatment?

I think we have achieved the highest level of technical proficiency, whatever the surgical approach may be, whether it be with well-trained surgeons in open surgery or in laparoscopic or robotic techniques. The reality is that some of the structures that course in the pelvis, including the two nerve bundles used for erections, will get traumatized. That is true. None of these surgical techniques, however, is truly superior to the other based on any data that I have seen about men getting their erections back in any more rapid fashion. Data, for instance, do not affirm the contention that laparoscopic or robotic surgery results in better or more rapidly recovered sexual function than highly qualified open surgery. The fact is that it may take a year or more for nerves to recover their function with any surgical technique.

In the meantime, can we develop medical therapies that can be based on better understanding with what is going on with the nerve trauma? Can we understand these injuries any better? This is a matter of discovering how the nerves can start once again to function. How to make these nerves be more functional. They are preserved in nerve sparing; however, after surgery, they are just not that functional. And currently they need time from their being traumatized to regain function. Many men say, "I don't want to get diagnosed, and I don't want to be treated because of the aftereffects, and I won't be a man anymore. I am not functional with this or that." That's why they don't want to be screened: because they fear what's going to happen to them. So that's the underlying basis of why I think we have to develop better treatments and achieve better outcomes. Some men aren't even worried whether they will lose their erections and/or whether they will lose urinary control.

But as physicians, we always recognize the big perspective. Our goal is first to make sure we save your life. Then preserve urinary control. And then preserve erectile function. Any other order doesn't make any kind of sense if you are a person who values life. But if the common perception out there is, "If I pursue treatment I'll definitely endure complications," you can see how people run away from being properly diagnosed. So what I think is the important objective still to be met—talking about the future of treatment being better—is that the ever-important area and the theme of my research at Johns Hopkins is, what are the ways we can improve the nerve function recovery? Currently, we are advancing some novel ideas toward developing therapies that would make nerve recovery better and faster.

What has been our progress in dealing with advanced cancer, and what can we look forward to in the future?

Prostate cancer presents itself early and late. When it is late, there is not a great deal that can be done. That is the tragedy for these men. The course of their treatment will almost certainly be palliative, not curable. We are counting on awareness to keep their numbers down. It is increasingly rare that you see these patients showing up on our doorstep with a PSA of 100 or more, but sometimes we do see it. Other than that, the most sobering situation in advanced cancer are the guys who we think, "We're on time with their treatment for suspected localized disease," but whose cancer progresses because of its aggressiveness. For example, with Gleason scores of 8 to 10. Their disease is found to have spread microscopically even though they may already have been administered a prostatectomy or radiation therapy. This is determined by PSA levels that do not remain at unmeasurable levels after treatment. We have to conclude that they have cancer cells in the body, and they may be microscopic, too minimal yet for bone scans to pick it up as one of the indicators of disease recurrence. When prostate cancer spreads, it has a predilection for bones. That's one of the early places it goes besides lymph nodes and tissue.

So what do you do with those guys? Have they really chosen the holy grail with hormone suppressions? I don't think so. It just slows the progression, but it does not cure it. Do we yet have effective chemotherapy for prostate cancer? Many drugs are currently being studied, but so far no silver bullet has been found. I'd like to think that we will one day develop the chemo-therapies that rival what we've done when faced with a Lance Armstrong–type testicular cancer that has spread, or when some-body who has a leukemia may be saved for a long, long time. I think the frontier of dealing with advanced prostate cancer still needs to be explored. We haven't achieved it yet. And I think there needs to be continued investigation by medical oncologists working with scientists in addition to what surgeons are doing deal-ing with better treatments for surgery. We have not achieved the holy grail by any means in dealing with advanced prostate cancer. What are the molecular mechanisms associated with advanced prostate cancer that develops and proliferates? We need to have much better targeting of disease using chemotherapy.

Can prostate cancer really be prevented, or is that a high-flown concept?

My answer is that I believe we have to pay attention to the pre-vention of prostate cancer. There's a lot of attention not only to environment but also to diet. People ask, "Should I be supple-menting my diet with soybeans? Should I take selenium with tomato products?" I think all of these questions are important to consider. There's interest today in lycopene, the chemical sub-stance responsible for the red or pink colors in tomatoes and pink grapefruit. I don't think that trying to go on certain diets for pro-state cancer prevention is crazy, but I do think it's not yet well defined. According to studies by the National Cancer Institute and by Harvard University, the link between tomato products and prostate cancer is being extensively investigated. Results of the Harvard study showed that men who ate ten or more servings of tomatoes or tomato products a week lowered their risk of prostate cancer by 45 percent. The researchers indicated that lycopene is at least partly responsible for this benefit. Other trial stud-ies are under way to determine if vitamin E and selenium help lowering one's prostate cancer risk. It all falls back on what we understand about the epidemiology of prostate cancer. The incidence and prevalence in populations. The real deal is that pro-state cancer is prevalent in developed countries. Genetics may also play a role, but there may be some other factors in terms of diet and environment that are relevant. All of us are sitting around here considering improvements in other areas, but prevention of pro-state cancer is a very important area.

Prevention comes on two different levels: primary prevention and secondary prevention. Secondary means if you've been diag-nosed and treated, if you've been cured, what kind of steps can you take to be sure you don't get a recurrence? And if you've been treated, but it's not clear that you've truly been cured, what addi-tional things can you do? The bottom line is that we have been doing well in managing prostate cancer and our advances have been steady. But much more has to be accomplished. This is no time to rest on our laurels.

Resources

Prostate Cancer Information

American Cancer Society
(800) ACS-2345
www.cancer.org

*American Foundation for
    Urologic Diseases*
(866) RING-AUA
www.urologyhealth.org

Hospice Foundation of America
(305) 981-2522
www.hospicefoundation.org

*James Buchanan Brady
    Urological Institute*
600 North Wolfe Street
Baltimore, MD 21287-2101
(410) 955-6707
http://urology.jhu.edu

Krongrad Institute
2110 Biscayne Boulevard, Suite 208

Aventura, FL 33180
(305) 936-0474
www.laprp.com

*Memorial Sloan-Kettering
    Cancer Center*
1275 York Avenue
New York, NY 10065
(212) 639-2000; (800)
    525-2225
www.mskcc.org

National Cancer Institute
(800) 4 CANCER
www.cancer.gov

*National Hospice and Palliative
    Care Organization*
1700 Diagonal Road, Suite 625
Alexandria, VA 22314
(703) 837-1500
www.nho.org

Obediah Cole Foundation
  (for prostate cancer)
www.obcolefoundation.org

Phoenix5
www.phoenix5.org

Prostate Cancer Foundation
1250 Fourth Street
Santa Monica, CA 90401
(800) 757-2873
www.prostatecancerfoundation.org

Prostate Cancer and Gay Men
http://health.groups
  .yahoo.com/group/
    prostatecancerandgaymen/

Urinary Incontinence
www.malecontinence.com

Us TOO International
(630) 795-1002; Support Hotline
  (800) 808-7866
Fax (630) 795-2602
www.ustoo.com

Implants and Devices

American Medical Systems, Inc.
10700 Bren Road West
Minnetonka, MN 55343
(952) 930-6000; (800) 328-3881
Fax: (952) 930-6373
Designer and manufacturer of
  prosthetic devices for control of
  urinary incontinence and sexual
  dysfunction.

Vivus, Inc.
1172 Castro Street
Mountain View, CA 94040-5311
(650) 934-5200
www.vivus.com
Manufacturer of innovative
  therapies to address sexual
  health, including erectile
  dysfunction.

References

Foreword

Senator John Kerry's sources are drawn from the American Cancer Society, "Facts and Figures 2007–2008"; "Cancer Facts and Figures for African Americans 2007–2008"; National Cancer Institute, U.S. National Institutes of Health Web site, www.cancer.gov.

Introduction

American Cancer Society, "Facts and Figures 2007," www.cancer.org.

Bouchardy, C., et al. "Recent trends in prostate cancer mortality show a continuous decrease in several countries." *Canary Journal*, August 31, 2008.

Scardino, Peter, and Judith Kelman. *Dr. Peter Scardino's Prostate Book*. New York: Avery, 2005.

U.S. National Cancer Institute, U.S. National Institutes of Health, www.cancer.gov. Prostate cancer statistical update, 2008.

Walsh, Patrick C., and Janet Ferrar Worthington. *Dr. Patrick Walsh's Guide to Surviving Prostate Cancer*, 1st ed. New York: Warner, 2001.

_____. *Dr. Patrick Walsh's Guide to Surviving Prostate Cancer*, 2nd ed. New York: Warner Wellness, 2007.

Other

Alterowitz, Ralph, and Barbara Alterowitz. *Intimacy with Impotence*. Cambridge, MA: Life Long, 2004.

Ellsworth, Pamela, John Heaney, and Cliff Gill. *100 Questions & Answers about Prostate Cancer*. Sudbury, MA: Jones and Barlett, 2003.

Survivors of Prostate Cancer

Below is a list of well-known survivors of prostate cancer.

Marion Barry

Harry Belafonte

Robert De Niro

Senator Christopher Dodd

Senator Bob Dole

Rudy Giuliani

Phil Lesh

Nelson Mandela

Roger Moore

General Colin Powell

General H. Norman Schwarzkopf

Frank Sinatra Jr.

Joe Torre

Bishop Desmond Tutu

Index